The ANTI-ARTHRITIS DIET

Increase Mobility and Reduce Pain with This 28-Day Life-Changing Program

JOSEPH KANDEL, M.D.
DAVID B. SUDDERTH, M.D.

PRIMA HEALTH
A Division of Prima Publishing

NUTRITIONAL ANALYSES: A per serving nutritional breakdown is provided for each recipe. If a range is given for an ingredient amount, the breakdown is based on the smaller number. If a range is given for servings, the breakdown is based on the larger number. If a choice of ingredients is given in an ingredient listing, the breakdown is calculated using the first choice. Nutritional content may vary depending on the specific brands or types of ingredients used. "Optional" ingredients or those for which no specific amount is stated are not included in the breakdown. Nutritional figures are rounded to the nearest whole number.

DISCLAIMER: This book is not meant to be a substitute for medical counseling or a guide for those on restricted diets. Readers with restricted diets should follow the guidance of their physician. The author and Prima Publishing shall have neither liability nor responsibility to any person or entity with respect to any loss, damage, or injury caused or alleged to be caused directly or indirectly by the information contained in this book.

Thanks to the Ralph Lauren Polo Store at the Waterside Shops in Naples, Florida, for the place settings and flatware used on the cover.

Library of Congress Cataloging-in-Publication Data

Kandel, Joseph.
The anti-arthritis diet: increase mobility and reduce pain with this 28-day life-changing program/Joseph Kandel. David B. Sudderth.
p. cm.
Includes index.
ISBN 0-7615-1260-8
1. Arthritis—Diet therapy. I. Sudderth, David B. II. Title.
RC933.A2K36 1998
616.7'220654—dc21 98-4604
CIP

98 99 00 01 DD 10 9 8 7 6 5 4 3 2 1
Printed in the United States of America

How to Order
Single copies may be ordered from Prima Publishing, P.O. Box 1260BK, Rocklin, CA 95677; telephone (916) 632-4400. Quantity discounts are also available. On your letterhead, include information concerning the intended use of the books and the number of books you wish to purchase.

Visit us online at www.primahealth.com

To all of my teachers and physician mentors who have trained me to learn how to learn, to think for myself, and never to stop caring. And to my patients, who remind me each and every day why I love medicine. But most of all, this book is dedicated to my father, the brightest and most caring man I have ever known.

JOSEPH

For Mai Lea

DAVID

Contents

Acknowledgments

TO BELLA KANDEL, FOR HER PROOFREADING OF THE recipes and all of her helpful comments during the preparation of this manuscript.

To Merry, Max, Hannah, and Geena, for taste-testing the meals and providing helpful and insightful comments!

To Mai Lea, for her tireless assistance in entering all of the information to obtain the nutritional assessment of the meals.

JOSEPH KANDEL, MD
DAVID B. SUDDERTH, MD

Introduction

FOOD CAN ACT AS MEDICINE, OR, AS THE OLD SAYING goes, "You are what you eat." Indeed, it is not only stroke, heart attack, diabetes, or your cholesterol level that merit diet attention and modification. Rather, it is also very true that when it comes to arthritis, you are profoundly impacted by what you eat. Why? Because some foods can cause your joints to become angry and inflamed.

In this book we explain the basics of arthritis—because, after all, that's what got you to pick up this book in the first place. We also explain the basic do's and don'ts of nutrition, and our view that concentrating on cutting calories may not be the sole answer in your quest for a healthful lifestyle and a healthy body.

We are not the food police, nor are we extremists in our beliefs, but we have provided some relatively strict guidelines for eating. With our tempting and delicious selections of twenty-eight breakfasts, twenty-eight lunches, and twenty-eight dinners, we demonstrate how easy it is to start yourself on your journey to a new you: healthier, more fit, and less painful. And of course, as if that weren't enough, we also introduce you to nutritious snacks that can keep you from going off of this diet when you just have to have "a little something."

Holidays invariably loom up before you're ready to face them. How do you go about staying on your healthy diet, ensuring that you don't affect more than your waistline? Why, you can prepare our healthful holiday meals. These recipes are perfect for entertaining friends and family, or for eating any time in a festive yet nutritious and healthy fashion.

Sometimes, diet is not enough and supplements are in order. As a result, we've outlined our own views and rationale towards approaching this very complex subject. When it comes to supplements, any text on arthritis would be incomplete if it didn't discuss the natural ingredients glucosamine and chondroitan sulfate. While we have discussed them in prior books, particularly *The Arthritis Solution,* now we have even more experience, as well as anecdotal cures that we thought you would like to read about.

Finally, this book is about living a healthy lifestyle, not just eating a healthy diet. For this reason, we've included a section on proper lifestyle activities, and explained how what you eat and how you live affects your arthritis and how you feel. Your frame of mind is a major player in your appreciation of the world around you. If you are hurting already, a negative attitude can sometimes amplify your pain. We provide healthful hints to alleviate some of this suffering from your chronic arthritis pain. These suggestions, combined with exercise, a healthy lifestyle, and a healthy diet, can launch you on your journey to a new you, a healthier you, a pain-free you.

Enjoy!

Joseph Kandel, MD
David B. Sudderth, MD
Chef Neal O'Hara

THE 28-DAY DIET

Week One	Breakfast	Lunch	Dinner
Monday	Indian Breakfast	Chicken Soup with Wild Rice	Winter Vegetable Roast
Tuesday	Far East Omelet	Portabella Mushroom and Spinach Sandwich	Grilled Chicken with Garlic
Wednesday	Spicy Johnny Cakes	Calamari Salad	Grilled Lamb Chop with Braised Red Cabbage
Thursday	Scrambled Egg White with Shiitake Mushroom and White Asparagus	Beef and Pasta Soup	Baked Pork Chops with Apples and Prunes
Friday	Spiced Granola and Yogurt	Chicken Orange Salad	Baked Salmon with Orange Sauce
Saturday	Egg White Frittata with Salsa	Citrus Salad	Savoy Cabbage with Salmon
Sunday	Egg White French Toast	Cabbage and Noodles	Moroccan Chicken with Rice

Week Two	Breakfast	Lunch	Dinner
Monday	Multigrain Prune Muffins	Seared Snapper Sandwich	Stuffed Pork Tenderloin with Fruit
Tuesday	Turkey Sausage Patty	Tuna Couscous Salad	Broiled Salmon over Greens with Pumpkin Seed Vinaigrette
Wednesday	Natural Breakfast Cereal	Turkey Burger on Pita	Ginger Sesame Chicken and Pasta Salad
Thursday	Breakfast Smoothie	Spinach Crepes	Chicken in Orange Sauce
Friday	Broiled Grapefruit	Chicken Pizza	Tuna Wrapped in Cabbage over Couscous
Saturday	Oatmeal Pancakes with Mixed Berry Sauce	Spinach Salad	Lemon Honey Ginger Chicken
Sunday	Stacked Waffles	Spinach Lasagna	Cinnamon-seared Sea Bass

THE 28-DAY DIET

Week Three	Breakfast	Lunch	Dinner
Monday	ADA	Red Beans and Rice with Pork Tenderloin	Grilled Monkfish with Spice Rub and Fruit
Tuesday	Breakfast Leeks	Tuna Honduran	Crunchy Chicken with Lemon Curry Sauce
Wednesday	Baked Apples	Roast Chicken Salad with Pineapple and Curry Vinaigrette	Spinach Salmon
Thursday	Chilled Fresh Fruit Breakfast Soup	Indian Chicken Salad	Grilled Tuna with Mango Salsa
Friday	Baked Banana with Granola and Mango	Blood Orange and Walnut Salad	Ostrich with Figs and Cranberries
Saturday	Rice Water	Pasta and Asparagus	Pork with Cherry Sauce over Polenta
Sunday	Blueberry-Banana Muffins	Roast Pork Tenderloin on Mixed Greens with Pear Vinaigrette	Caramelized Salmon with Melon Sauce

Week Four	Breakfast	Lunch	Dinner
Monday	Poor Man's Pudding	Grilled Monkfish, Fennel, and Parsnips with Honduran Cabbage	Baked Chicken with Wild Rice
Tuesday	Breakfast Salad	Three-Green, Citrus, Walnut, and Banana Salad	Citrus Chicken
Wednesday	Blueberry Bagel	Root Vegetable Salad	Baked Turkey Cutlets
Thursday	Rice with Fruit	Pumpkin Seed Salad	Spinach Eggplant Pizza
Friday	Cold Cantaloupe	Jicama Salad	Seared Pompano and Salsa Cruda with Polenta
Saturday	Fried Polenta with Mixed Berries	Vegetable and Pasta Bouillabaisse	Poached Turkey with Wild Mushrooms
Sunday	Consommé with Lemon and Angel Hair	Roast Vegetable Sandwich	Home-cured Salmon

Chapter 1

WHAT IS OSTEOARTHRITIS?

ARTHRITIS IS AN EXTREMELY PERVASIVE DISEASE: IT affects the rich and famous as well as the poor and unknown worldwide. About 40 million Americans have some form of osteoarthritis, one of the most common human afflictions and the most common cause of disability in the United States. Arthritis does not discriminate. It strikes men and women and even children of all races. Arthritis affects the same joints in men and women until we reach our mid-fifties. As women age, they tend to have more arthritis problems related to knees and hands, while men are more likely to experience the pain and stiffness of hip disease. Of course, both men and women can have arthritic problems anywhere they have joints in their bodies. Older Americans are the most long-suffering: X-ray studies reveal that as many as 70 percent of people over age sixty-five have a problem with arthritis.

WHEN YOU SEE IT AND HEAR IT—AND FEEL IT

Arthritis may begin silently, but eventually it makes itself known. Sometimes you see various types of deformities because of the proliferation of the bones. *Heberden's nodes* in the finger joints are very prominent, especially in women. These nodes affect the joints near the fingernails. The gross deformities of advanced hip arthritis are known to most physicians.

You can also hear arthritis as it advances. As bone rubs against bone, you hear a crackling sound (*crepitus*), not quite as bad as fingernails on a blackboard, but somewhat similar. This sound can also occur when the doctor places his or her hand on the joint in question during motion.

You may also feel a mild sensation of warmth over your arthritic joint. This is because the muscles that move and stabilize the arthritic joint may be smaller in bulk and shrink along the length of the muscle.

No specific blood test can help diagnosis arthritis, but the X-ray findings are fairly characteristic. The bone surfaces of the affected joint will tend to be closer together and you will see bone spurs that can become quite prominent. The doctor can also see areas of abnormal calcification immediately under the surface of the bone (*subchondral cysts*).

Only the most fortunate of us will escape some symptoms of arthritis in our lifetime. Pretty depressing, right? Not entirely. Because, unlike past generations, we are living in an age when much can be done about this primordial scourge. You *can* take action to stop your arthritis from getting any worse, and maybe even improve your condition. So read on!

WHAT IS ARTHRITIS?

Osteoarthritis is a debilitating and painful disease affects joints and bones in one or two areas or in numerous parts of the body. Also (mistakenly) known as "degenerative joint disease," it is primarily a disease of the cartilage that forms the articular surfaces of your joints. How does this damage start? It may have one or more causes:

- An injury to the joint by trauma—something falls on the joint and damages it.
- An injury stemming from inflammatory process—something causes the joint to swell up and arthritis subsequently develops.
- An abnormal stress on the joint.
- A genetic predisposition to arthritis.

As the arthritis progresses, the cartilage becomes more damaged, leading to significant pain and stiffness and sometimes disability and great difficulty using the diseased joint. The disease continues in a negative downward spiral unless the person takes proactive steps to halt and improve the process—actions that we recommend in this book and in our first book, *The Arthritis Solution.* No matter how you contracted arthritis, there are many things you can do to improve your condition. One way is by eating foods that help alleviate arthritis and avoiding those that make the problem worse. This, of course, is why we wrote this book and are offering you delicious recipes to try.

The Impact of Trauma on Your Joints

How can you traumatize a joint? The trauma can be physical, such as a bone fracture. If you fracture your ankle, for example, you will almost certainly eventually develop arthritis of the ankle. If you injure the ligaments of your knee, specifically the *meniscus* or *cruciate* ligaments, then you are going to develop arthritis in your wounded knee.

Eat foods that can alleviate your arthritis, and avoid those foods that make the problem worse.

An Inflammatory Process

Arthritis may be biochemically induced by your own body. Such is the case with gout, a form of arthritis that causes swelling and pain. Poorly managed gout (you don't take your medicine) and other metabolic joint diseases are also likely to ultimately develop into secondary arthritis.

Abnormal Stress on the Joints

Athletes know that the frequent, repetitive and forceful motions of the joints in tennis, running, and many other sports maneuvers can lead to arthritis. We see this in boxers who develop arthritis of the wrist and hands, and ballet dancers who develop arthritis of the ankle. You don't have to be an athlete to have this problem: Jackhammer operators, meat cutters, and people in a variety of other trades often develop arthritis in the joints from repetitive movements.

Carrying too much body weight may also lead to arthritis, or make your condition worse. Think about it: Your ankles, knees, and hips are often called on to bear your entire body weight. Add to that the force exerted on these joints during high-impact activities like such as jogging and jumping, and you can see the problem. Also, the "obese lifestyle" is an inactive one—inactivity is anathema to healthy joints. Arthritis really "loves" unhealthy joints.

Heredity and Environment

Genes also exert some control over the development of arthritis. In fact, researchers have identified specific genetic markers for certain types of arthritis. If your parents, brothers, or sisters have arthritis, then your risk is definitely elevated. While you cannot change your genes in your kitchen, you can change the size of your jeans there! Even the loss of a few pounds can lead to far less stress on your joints.

UNDERSTANDING THE HUMAN JOINT

To understand your illness, you need a little basic anatomy information. Learning about healthy and unhealthy joints in health and disease empowers us to adopt healthy lifestyle changes and take various other steps that lead to promoting health in these quite remarkable structures.

Unquestionably, joints are architectural and biological marvels. In mechanics, a joint is simply an attachment that allows two adjacent structures to move independently. The "design specifications" on a biological joint, however, are much more complex. For example, unlike a hardware hinge, a human joint is composed of living, breathing tissue. Live tissues need an opportunity to obtain nutrients and other necessary supplies metabolically and to rid themselves of subsequent waste products. That's where cartilage comes in.

There are no blood vessels in the *cartilage,* the most important component of the human joint, to ferry these supplies back and forth. Oxygen and other necessary chemicals simply circulate through the joint when you move. The cartilage functions as a sponge, compressing and relaxing, allowing necessary substances into the tissues and expelling breakdown products at the same time. Cartilage also has no nerve endings. This is why, despite carrying massive weight, no pain signals arrive at the brain.

Cartilage is a very common tissue in the human body. It supplies the "skeleton" for large portions of the human nose and ears, and plays a vital part in the health of your joints. Let's take a closer look.

Cartilage: Nature's Common Wonder

Cartilage is composed of a group of cells we call *chondrocytes,* and the cartilage matrix is comprised of water and some very large molecules. Water content of the cartilage matrix can reach up to 80 percent. The large molecules that comprise the majority of the remaining cartilage matrix include collagen and proteoglycans.

Collagen is a very tough and complex protein that is used in many parts of the body and confers strength and resilience. It is braided and entwined with other tissues in a complicated manner to allow cartilage, bone, and connective tissue to work together as a team to resist injury and maintain shape.

Proteoglycans are also quite large molecules. They are composed only partly of protein. Large numbers of sugar molecules are attached in a large, matted network of sponge-like consistency, which promotes a spring-like action and fiercely holds onto the surrounding water molecules.

Chondrocytes are cells that are dispersed in large numbers throughout the cartilage matrix. The chondrocytes not only form the large molecules discussed above, but they also release chemicals that are responsible for the breakdown of aging components of the cartilage matrix.

When you think about how many times a day you move your joints, you can see that cartilage is very active tissue. Proper health of the cartilage and the joint itself depends on a delicate balance of production of healthy joint components and retirement of the worn-out elements.

Other Important Structures of Your Joints

Other structures help maintain the proper structures of the joint itself. These include the joint capsule, the synovial membrane, and the ligaments, muscles, tendons, and bursae.

The *joint capsule* is a tubular structure that attaches to the ends of both bones forming the joint. The joint capsule is very tough, and it works to seal the joint from the external tissues.

Lining the inside of the joint capsule is the *synovial membrane*. This very sensitive structure secretes a slippery substance known as synovial fluid. When lubricated with the synovial fluid, the two ends of the joint cartilage can move against each other with only a fraction of the resistance present when two pieces of ice are rubbed together.

The joints are further stabilized by *ligaments,* both inside and outside the joint, as well as by *muscles* and their attachments, *tendons. Bursae,* small sacs similar to joints, lie immediately under the skin over bony prominences, allowing joints and bones to move under the skin without causing injury to the skin itself.

WHAT CAUSES ARTHRITIS?

Although we do know some causes of arthritis, we don't know all the reasons why some people suffer greatly, some a little, and others not at all. In some cases arthritis may have a profoundly significant genetic basis, while other cases seem to be a clear consequence of injury. For the vast majority of arthritis cases, there is no well-documented or understood cause.

That does not mean that every theory is conjecture. We suspect that the development of arthritis is primarily an issue of maintenance.

A Joint Is Like a Factory

Let's compare the cartilage in your joints to raw materials in a well-functioning factory. A factory needs raw materials and must also rid itself of waste products. Aging equipment must be maintained daily and replaced when necessary.

A similar maintenance process applies to human joints. Raw materials (oxygen and other nutrients) must be obtained and delivered to the chondrocytes, where they are fabricated into the cartilage matrix. The chondrocytes not only produce the major chemicals of the cartilage matrix; they also produce the elements of the destruction of worn-out tissue.

What Causes the Initial Problem?

We can't always identify the initial event that leads to the cascade of developing arthritis. But we do know that early on there is some water loss and also some thickening in the cartilage, an apparent response of the cartilage to protect itself. (It's ironic that as the body tries to protect itself, it starts a chain of events leading to further damage.)

Eventually, the cartilage softens, as a consequence of the poor quality of the hastily formed components of the cartilage matrix, which are lacking in structural integrity. This is somewhat like hiring someone to do a rush job on your roof repair because you have a major problem. The person does a slapdash job, which may later cause you more problems when the rainy season comes.

As a result of the change in consistency of the cartilage, small rips appear. These tears ultimately deepen and extend to the bone. The chondrocytes then tend to increase their numbers to make a final attempt to repair the damage, just as road repair crews slap more and more concrete on top of a pothole.

Changes that ultimately occur in the bone underneath the cartilage become extremely smooth and have an appearance of ivory (*eburnation*). The bone begins building up, which leads to formation of bone spurs (*osteophytes*). With these changes come visible deformities of the joints, and the sufferer may experience severe pain that leads to inactivity and further acceleration of this entire pathologic process.

And There's More!

As the process continues, we see a thickening of the synovial lining. Sometimes we also see inflammation in the synovial fluid itself. These various processes converge, causing increasing pain, stiffness, and loss of range of motion. The joint capsule thickens and the victim is left with a painful and basically useless joint. The deformity of the joints themselves then results in instability, which acts to further accelerate the arthritic process.

WHY DOES IT HURT SO MUCH IN THE MORNING?

You may wake up to pain in the morning and wonder why you're hurting, since you haven't done anything except sleep. You may wonder if you could be like one of those characters in the fairy tale about the sisters who danced all night until their shoes fell off. Discomfort related to arthritis is frequently described as a deep, aching sensation in the joint area. Nighttime pain is particularly common in the hip joint. You may have been asleep, but you feel like you worked—or danced—all night! Why?

The reason is simple. Arthritic pain is aggravated by non-use, and somewhat relieved by getting up and moving about.

Where Does the Pain Come From?

If there are no actual nerve fibers in the joint cartilage itself, why does it hurt? Because there are plenty of pain-sensitive structures in and about the joint itself. For example, the synovial membrane often becomes inflamed, which in turn leads to production of chemicals that irritate pain-sensitive nerve fibers.

The bone underneath the cartilage is also quite sensitive to pain—particularly when there are small fractures, which complicate advanced arthritis. As *osteophytes* (bone spurs) develop, they attempt to stretch your very pain-sensitive *periosteum* (membrane overlying all bones). Bone spurs can also press on nearby tissues, such as tendons, ligaments, and nerves, which can ultimately lead to severe pain that radiates far away from the actual site of irritation.

The joint capsules can also become inflamed and stretched and the muscles surrounding the arthritic joint may reflexively contract in an involuntary spasm as an involuntary protective mechanism to halt movement of the painful joint. In trying to protect itself, your body is again causing you more pain and more problems.

Progressive joint deterioration can cause other symptoms outside the joint itself, as we mentioned above. Bone spurs in the spine can cause a radiating pain from the neck into the arm or low back pain radiating into the leg (sciatica).

Arthritis of the wrist with tendinitis can lead to pinched nerves at the wrist (carpal tunnel syndrome), which can cause not only painful symptoms in the hands but also numbness, weakness, and loss of control. Arthritis of the spine can cause injury to the spinal cord and nerves within the spinal canal. Arthritis of the upper cervical (neck portion) spine can cause severe headaches that often respond to conventional treatment of arthritis rather than conventional treatment of tension headaches or migraines.

NORMAL PHYSICAL ACTIVITY IS GOOD

Exercise—along with the healthy diet outlined in this book—is the cornerstone in prevention and treatment of arthritis.

This doesn't mean that if you have arthritis you should lie down or become a couch potato. Not a good choice at all! The usual athletic activities such as walking or jogging are not risk factors for arthritis.

Studies of middle-aged joggers have shown no increase of arthritis of the knees or hips when compared to non-joggers. This leads us to a very simple, yet supremely important conclusion: *Exercise does not cause arthritis.* Actually, exercise—along with the healthy diet outlined in this book—is the cornerstone in prevention and treatment of arthritis.

Read on!

Chapter 2

WHAT'S FOOD GOT TO DO WITH IT?

IT'S TRUE: WHAT YOU CONSUME DIRECTLY AFFECTS many aspects of your life, and one of those aspects is your arthritis. Never underestimate the power of diet! Dietary factors are implicated in virtually every modern disease: Parkinson's disease, Alzheimer's disease, diabetes, stroke, heart disease, cancer, some infections, and, of course, arthritis. New evidence indicates that some foods can actually alleviate your arthritis, while other foods can make it worse.

Never under-estimate the power of diet!

Evidence indicates that some foods can actually alleviate your arthritis, while other foods can make it worse.

How do you determine the best foods and dietary elements to control your arthritis—especially when we are bombarded nearly daily with newspaper or magazine articles offering melodramatic revelations of (supposedly) powerful new therapeutic agents that promise miraculous cures to many diseases? Despite the sensationalist claims that vie for our attention, there are many serious and clear voices with potent messages about the importance of diet for arthritis sufferers. In this chapter we'll provide you with the guidance you need.

FOOD IS MEDICINE

Most people realize that some foods we eat can clog arteries and ultimately lead to stroke or heart disease. But what most people do *not* know is that what we eat may also prevent this process. In an intriguing article reported in the *Journal of American Medical Association,* Dr. Gary Plotnik described how antioxidant vitamins can protect the interior lining of arteries (*endothelium*) from the ferocious fats trying to take over the walls of our blood vessels.

Even in healthy individuals with normal cholesterol levels, just one single fatty meal can neutralize our first line of defense (the endothelium) and lead to atherosclerosis (hardening of the arteries). This process, in turn, may lead to stroke, heart disease, and other problems.

Amazingly, the "endothelial paralysis" problem was blocked by pre-treatments before a fatty meal with the powerful antioxidant vitamins A and C. The final significance of this fascinating study is yet unknown. But it demonstrates the enormous power of how what we eat affects our health on both sides of the disease equation—contracting disease and avoiding it. Make no mistake: Food is medicine!

The same oxidative stress (see below) that is destroying your arteries also has its sights on the cartilage in your joints. We'll discuss the important subject of antioxidants in more detail later in this chapter. But they are not the only dietary influences on arthritis. For example, we know that vitamin D can slow the progression of arthritis. Even *not* eating has a significant effect. Fasting can also lead to a real improvement in acute aggravation of rheumatoid arthritis. However, we don't advocate starving yourself!

Weight loss alone can reduce the steady progression of arthritis, and not just by reducing the physical strain on your body. Potent biochemical processes are also at work in destroying the joints of the obese. Fortunately, as you'll see later in this chapter in Chapter 9, nutrients in some seafood and sea vegetables can beat up on the very powerful inflammatory mediating cells, that is, the neutrophils, which are key link in the inflammatory cascade. Fresh ginger can also help remove inflammatory symptoms in some individuals. (But be careful: Ginger can thin the blood and should be used with caution.) Other spices with reported anti-inflammatory properties include turmeric, cloves, and yucca.

FAT: A MORE BALANCED APPROACH

A fascinating article on diet and arthritis in *The Journal of American Veterinary Medicine Association* presented an intriguing report on the effect of diet on the development of arthritis. Forty-eight Labrador retrievers were followed over a five-year period. Half the dogs had unrestricted access to food, while the other group was only allowed to eat 75 percent of what their gluttonous cohorts were allowed.

So what happened? The dogs with the restricted diets showed dramatically less hip arthritis than the group allowed to eat all they wanted. Similar studies have been done on other species. In short, whether you lope, crawl, or ambulate in an erect bipedal manner, this diet thing is important!

CASE HISTORY:

A busy 43-year-old physician managed to gain approximately fifty pounds over a ten-year period. Long office hours and little time for exercise had taken its toll. Pasta diets and other dietary modifications were not helpful as the weight just kept piling on. Unfortunately, he had a family history of early osteoarthritis and his mother and her brother had both had hip replacements at a fairly early age. As the weight increased so did the hip pain. In the beginning it was just in the mornings but in time began to be prominent after periods of sitting, walking, or other activities. Exercise became difficult. By following the dietary recommendations presented in this book and exercising, he was able to reduce his weight by forty pounds over a six-month period. As the weight normalized the hip pain evaporated. He is now able to jog and is considering participating in an upcoming triathlon.

Some relationship between the consumption of fat and atherosclerosis has been recognized since the early twentieth century. Various groups of people and their diseases were compared with their eating habits. For example, a fatty diet could (and did) give monkeys heart attacks. These findings, combined with research from many animal experiments, established in the minds of many researchers and other influential individuals that fat was bad.

The impact of those animal experiments on the scientific community was dramatic. Dietary fat was demonized and the word rang out to the populace to slash their fat intake to 30 percent of the overall diet. Many people adopted these recommendations. As a result, we now eat more carbohydrates and less fat. Unfortunately, two decades later, Americans are fatter than ever. It didn't work.

The French Paradox

As aggravating as the French can be to helpless tourists on the streets of Paris, they really get annoying when it comes to coronary heart disease. Why? Because despite the fact that the French consumption patterns of dietary fats are similar to those in the United States (as are their patterns for high blood pressure, cigarette smoking, and so on), people in France have a much lower coronary heart disease rate than individuals living in the United States. In fact, the rate of heart disease in the United States is more than twice that of France.

Why? Bioflavonoids (we'll discuss these more later in this chapter) are thought by many to be responsible. It may also be true that the average French person's regular consumption of red wine may be the answer to this dilemma. Alcohol in moderation can then be a benefit. It is clear that large amounts of alcohol can affect essentially all tissues including the brain and muscle. Alcohol-induced muscle weakness leads to joint instability and further joint deterioration.

While we do not recommend alcohol in large quantities, we feel that it would be almost sinful not to enjoy a glass of red wine with some of the wonderful recipes we present in this book!

We feel that the extreme adjustments in America's diet have been a mistake. The fat scare failed miserably in terms of reducing the obesity epidemic. More than 30 percent of us are fatter than we were just two short decades ago. A more detailed discussion of these matters would go beyond the scope of the present work, and for this reason we would recommend the excellent discussion found in Dr. Barry Sears' book *Enter The Zone*.

We fully agree that some fats are best left alone or greatly reduced. But all fats are not equal; what's important is the category of fat. When considering the importance of a specific type of fat, we feel it's best to approach the issue on a case-by-case basis. First, let's talk about some different kinds of fat.

Saturated Fatty Acids

Saturated fatty acids are the type of fat found in dairy and meat products. They tend to increase bad cholesterol (LDL) and increase the risk of atherosclerosis and blood clots. Reducing this fat in your diet tends to lower total and LDL cholesterol.

Mono-unsaturated Fatty Acids

Olive oil and rape seed (canola) oil belong in the mono-unsaturated fatty acid category. In Mediterranean countries, where these oils are frequently used, there appears to be a lower incidence of some types of cancer as well as of atherosclerosis. And people live longer! These are the cooking oils that we recommend.

Trans Fatty Acids

Whoa! This is the really bad stuff. These are fats produced artificially to make cooking oils like margarine and shortening more solid and less likely to become rancid. You will find these in cakes, biscuits, and other baked goods containing margarine or partially hydrogenated (solid) vegetable shortening. Trans fatty acids influence good and bad cholesterol both in the wrong direction. There may be no cholesterol in your margarine, yet your bad cholesterol goes up anyway. Check labels of foods you buy. If you see the words "partially hydrogenated," stay away!

Polyunsaturated Fatty Acids

Polyunsaturated fatty acids are very important dietary constituents that cannot be made by the human body. They come in two types: Omega 6 and Omega 3. We have a lot to say about them later in this chapter.

Olestra

Olestra is a fat substitute introduced by the snack food industry. The Food and Drug Administration (FDA) now requires all products containing Olestra to state the following: "Olestra may cause abdominal cramping and loose stools."

A recent article in the Journal of the American Medical Association suggests that the gastrointestinal side effects of Olestra are probably exaggerated. In a study, 1,123 volunteers consumed either Olestra-containing potato chips or standard potato chips. After one sitting, there was no difference in the amount of diarrhea or other gastrointestinal symptoms between the groups. The precise consequences of this study are unclear at this point, although they suggest, at least in modest amounts, Olestra is not as hard on the GI tract as some people contend. We are adopting a wait-and-see position on Olestra for now.

"Fat" Pills: Good or Bad?

The Food and Drug Administration withdrew Redux and Pondimin on September 5, 1997, due to reports in the *New England Journal of Medicine* that suggested serious cardiac-related effects of these medications. Complaints included elevated pressure in the circulation of the lungs (pulmonary hypertension) and disease of the cardiac valves.

New drugs for weight loss have been developed. In 1997, the FDA approved two new weight loss agents: Meridia™ and Xenical™. Meridia (sibutramine hydrochloride monohydrate) capsules have been developed by Knolo Pharmaceuticals. The company launched this drug for weight loss and maintaining weight loss, along with a lifestyle modified program to include reduced calorie diet as well as exercise. Meridia apparently affects appetite-regulating chemicals (neurotransmitters) such as serotonin. Meridia prevents serotonin from being reabsorbed from cells and thus it makes more of these substances functionally available. It will be taken once a day.

Studies have indicated that the drugs also help overweight individuals who suffer from high blood pressure. The medication has been tested on 6,000 patients. Meridia does have some apparently mild side effects, including sleep difficulties, constipation, headache, and dry mouth. Rarely, the drug can increase blood pressure. It is not recommended for individuals who have a history of poorly controlled blood pressure, congestive heart failure, stroke, or significant coronary artery disease. Premarketing studies have not demonstrated the pulmonary hypertension and valvular disease that were found in earlier weight-reducing agents such as Redux.

Xenical (Orlistat) is the first of a new class of weight-controlling medications. This medication doesn't enter the brain or affect the appetite. Instead, it works by controlling the amount of fats absorbed from the intestine. Swedish studies have indicated that obese individuals lost approximately 10 percent of their body weight, and they actually keep the weight off. The weight loss was attended by improvement in parameters related to cholesterol, blood pressure and glucose/insulin.

By blocking the enzymes (biologic catalysts) that break down fat in the intestine, the fat will continue through the intestine and be discharged with the stool. This drug is proposed to treat obese individuals on a long-term basis. No serious medical side effects have been reported.

Some critics of Xenical are concerned that it could interfere with the absorption of many vital components of our diet including antioxidants, especially vitamins A and E. Unless some unexpected side effects result from this medication, we suspect this medication will be a commercial success. We are excited by these new agents but will definitely not be the first doctors on the block to be recommending these to our overweight patients.

YES! WE STILL NEED CARBOHYDRATES

Carbohydrates are extremely important, and we do not want to eliminate them from our diet. Yet we think that the pendulum has swung much too far in favor of carbohydrates. We recommend that the carbohydrates you consume should be mostly in the form of complex carbohydrates: vegetables, legumes, whole grains, and fruit. Reduce the amounts of simple carbohydrates—refined sugars and simple starches, such as pasta, white bread, and white rice.

In our recipes we recommend certain substitutions on a regular basis: whole-grain flour and bread rather than refined white flour products, olive oil or canola oil for cooking, nonfat yogurt, and turbino, a raw, brown sugar, as a substitute sweetener for refined sugar.

ANTIOXIDANTS *VERSUS* FREE RADICALS

As oxygen is taken from the bloodstream into the tissues and metabolized in the course of energy production, a small portion of the oxygen forms both a highly reactive super-oxidant anion (O2-) and hydrogen peroxide. Hydrogen peroxide can freely enter all body cells as well as the smaller compartments of the cells. These and similar chemicals are known as *free radicals*.

Free radicals are very reactive and extremely unstable, existing typically only for a fraction of a second. Yet they can react with proteins as well as various other important structures, including our genetic material (DNA) to cause tissue damage implicated in a large array of medical problems: arthritis, atherosclerosis, some types of cancer, and many other diseases. Antioxidants, which include vitamins A, C, and E, as well as selenium, act as scavengers, neutralizing these highly reactive free radicals.

VITAMIN E

Vitamin E is one of the good guys. In addition to improving arthritis, vitamin E also seems to be helpful in reducing atherosclerosis. In one study of people who used vitamin E, their risk of heart attack was reduced by one-third.

There are four forms of vitamin E: alpha, beta, gamma, and delta tocopherols. The alpha type is the vitamin E found in your body, while gamma is vitamin E in foodstuffs. The alpha type of vitamin E is the usual type of vitamin E found commercially. At least one manufacturer produces a "mixed vitamin E."

Vitamin E also has an anti-clotting effect, which might affect people who are on blood-thinning medication. If you are on these medications, you should definitely discuss this with your doctor. Vitamin E is found in certain vegetables, such as sunflower seeds and their oil, avocados, peaches, broccoli, spinach, and asparagus. We recommend 200 to 800 International Units (IU) of vitamin E daily.

Vitamin A and the Carotenoids

These antioxidants are found in liver, milk, eggs, and liver oils from fish, such as cod and halibut. Other sources include colored fruits, such as orange, yellow, or red fruits and vegetables, as well as green leafy vegetables. Vitamin A can be taken in excess and can cause severe visual problems when taken in excess. The recommended daily dose of vitamin A is approximately 5,000 IU.

Vitamin C

Vitamin C is a very powerful antioxidant. It is of course found in many different types of fruit, including oranges, kiwi, papaya, and mango, as well as vegetables, such as potatoes.

Selenium

Selenium is an antioxidant obtained from various food sources as well as dietary supplements. The content of food grown in a particular area will vary in terms of its amount of selenium due to variation in local soil. Typically, meats, chicken, and seafood are sources of this antioxidant, as are grains and some nuts. The maximum amount of selenium recommended is 200 micrograms. Vitamin E interacts with selenium, making it more powerful and lessening the need for large amounts.

Vitamin D

A study reported in the *Annals of Internal Medicine* has suggested that low intake and low serum levels of vitamin D can accelerate the progression of osteoarthritis of the knee. This does not imply that arthritis is actually prevented by this vitamin, but merely that the rate of progression is decreased. Vitamin D requires sunlight to be activated to calciferol, the active form. Good sources of vitamin D include fatty fish (tuna, salmon, herring, sardines, mackerel), fish oils like halibut and cod liver, shrimp, cheese, milk fat, butter, egg yolk, and cereals.

FOODS THAT AFFECT INFLAMMATION

Most types of arthritis cause inflammation. It typically appears as pain, swelling, increased heat emission, and often redness. Inflammation is not only painful, it can also lead to tissue destruction. Chemicals called *prostaglandins* and *leukotriene* affect inflammation. What we eat can make the inflammation worse or better.

Omega 3 and Omega 6 Fatty Acids and Inflammation

As we said earlier, the polyunsaturated fats in our diet fall into two different categories: Omega 3 and Omega 6. These molecules form the raw material for prostaglandin and leukotriene synthesis. They fulfill important roles in the inflammatory response.

Omega 6—Ouch!

Our Western diet contains mostly the Omega 6 variety. (And guess which one is the bad one? Yup, Omega 6.) Omega 6 fats are present in a number of our food preparation products, including safflower, sunflower, and corn oils. These oils are converted to arachidonic acid, a major player in the initiation of the inflammatory process. Arachidonic acid is also found in egg yolks, red meat, high-fat dairy, and chicken products.

Omega 3—Ahhh!

Omega 3 oils are good, and increasing these substances can actually stop the inflammatory response. Omega 3s are present in fish oils, especially cold water fish such as salmon, mackerel, and tuna. Some vegetable oils, such as black currant, flaxseed, borage seed, and evening primrose, are also sources of Omega 3 oils. These fragile oils can be damaged by certain preparation practices, primarily deep-frying.

Bioflavonoids

Flavanoids fall within a group of over 20,000 compounds, and they appear to have remarkable health benefits. Flavonoids are essentially a group of plant pigments. In plants, they are protective from the harshness of the environment and the elements. In humans, these compounds act in a variety of healthy ways: as antiviral, antioxidant, anti-allergic, and—most important for us—anti-inflammatory. These free radical–gobbling agents seem to reduce the tendency of the blood to clot and appear to reduce the risk of cancer. They are also involved in maintaining healthy blood vessels and enhancing the effectiveness of vitamin C.

A 1995 study in the *Archives of Internal Medicine* demonstrated a reduced risk of heart disease in countries where bioflavonoids were commonly found in the diet. As noted earlier, the French paradox may very well be related to their consumption of bioflavonoids. Bioflavonoids are found in many fruits and vegetables, including onions, green beans, broccoli, celery, endive, cranberry, and kale.

Citrus fruits are particularly good sources of bioflavonoids, both the peel and the white pulp. Other sources include tea, red wine, lettuce, broad beans, tomatoes, red peppers, apples (especially in the peel), and strawberries. A potent sub-group of bioflavonoids is the *proanthocyanidines*. They are found in particularly brightly colored fruits and vegetables such as red, green, and yellow bell peppers, purple eggplant, pink grapefruit, and yellow squash.

Chapter 3

BREAKFAST

Your Fast, Delicious, and Nutritious Start to a Healthier Life

WE'VE ALL HEARD THE OLD ADAGE, "BREAKFAST IS THE most important meal of the day." If you plan to enjoy an energetic, healthy, positive, and exciting day, then breakfast is necessary.

Your body is like a finely tuned machine: It needs energy to run. Without that energy you'll suffer from decreased stamina, attention, and vim and vigor. Remember, breakfast comes from two words: break and fast. From the evening before until the next morning, it may be twelve or more hours from your last meal. You need to fill up your tank! And, like a high-performance automobile, what you put into your tank makes a difference. You can choose health, fitness, and a positive direction by starting your day with a healthy and nutritious meal that tastes good and is also good for you.

To enjoy an energetic, healthy, positive, and exciting day, then breakfast is necessary.

In this chapter we offer you thirty delicious breakfasts, taking into account that we don't always have time to make a gourmet meal in the morning. Nevertheless, you need to start yourself off on the right foot, and the right breakfast certainly can be the beginning to a healthy day. With breakfast, as with the other meals, we do want to point out that we are not the food police, nor do we intend to be extremists. We have taken some liberties in order to make starting and maintaining this anti-arthritis diet reasonable, relatively simple, and effective. If you want to start the day with a gourmet meal, you'll find recipes here. And if you just want a quick, easy, and nutritious start, you'll find that too. We hope you enjoy your healthy start and begin a journey to a healthier, more mobile, and less painful you. Enjoy!

Scrambled Egg White with Shiitake Mushroom and White Asparagus

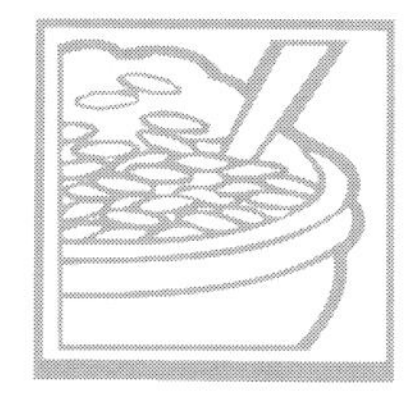

2 SERVINGS

3 white asparagus (or green, if white is unavailable), bottoms trimmed
1 tablespoon olive oil
1 tablespoon chopped shallots
3 shiitake mushrooms, fresh or dried, stems removed
2 egg whites, beaten
1 tablespoon chopped green onions

1. Blanche asparagus in boiling water for 1 minute. Refresh in ice cold water, drain, and set aside.

2. In a nonstick skillet, heat olive oil on medium heat. Sauté shallots and mushrooms until tender.

3. Swirl in eggs and green onion. Scramble until done. Top with asparagus.

PER SERVING
Calories 104
Calories from Fat 71
Percent Total Calories From:
Fat 69%
Protein 19%
Carbohydrates 13%
Percent RDA:
Vitamin A 17%
Vitamin C 14%
Calcium 0%
Iron 3%

Nutrient	Amount per Serving	% Daily Value
Total Fat	8 g	12%
Saturated Fat	1 g	5%
Cholesterol	0 mg	0%
Sodium	58 mg	2%
Total Carbohydrate	3 g	1%
Dietary Fiber	0 g	2%
Sugars	0 g	
Protein	5 g	

Blueberry Bagel

4 SERVINGS

2 blueberry bagels
½ cup blackberries, smashed
1 medium banana, smashed
¼ cup plain nonfat yogurt

1. Cut bagels in half and toast them.

2. Mix fruit and yogurt, and spread on the bagel. Garnish with cottage cheese and peaches, if desired.

PER SERVING
Calories 128
Calories from Fat 12
Percent Total Calories From:
Fat 10%
Protein 12%
Carbohydrates 78%
Percent RDA:
Vitamin A 1%
Vitamin C 11%
Calcium 0%
Iron 5%

Nutrient	Amount per Serving	% Daily Value
Total Fat	1 g	2%
Saturated Fat	0 g	2%
Cholesterol	2 mg	1%
Sodium	106 mg	4%
Total Carbohydrate	25 g	8%
Dietary Fiber	1 g	5%
Sugars	0 g	
Protein	4 g	

Breakfast Smoothie

6 SERVINGS

1 cup crushed ice
¼ cup plain nonfat yogurt
½ tablespoon honey
Pinch ground cinnamon
1½ cups chopped mixed fruit (mango, banana, strawberry, and so on)

1. In a blender, mix all ingredients together and blend until foamy. If too thick, thin out with fruit juice. If too thin, thicken with yogurt.

2. Garnish with sliced fruit and mint leaves.

PER SERVING
Calories 41
Calories from Fat 5
Percent Total Calories From:
Fat 11%
Protein 5%
Carbohydrates 84%
Percent RDA:
Vitamin A 0%
Vitamin C 3%
Calcium 0%
Iron 2%

Nutrient	Amount per Serving	% Daily Value
Total Fat	1 g	1%
Saturated Fat	0 g	1%
Cholesterol	1 mg	0%
Sodium	6 mg	0%
Total Carbohydrate	9 g	3%
Dietary Fiber	1 g	3%
Sugars	0 g	
Protein	1 g	

Oatmeal Pancakes with Mixed Berry Sauce

10 SERVINGS

1⅛ cups nonfat milk
1 cup rolled oats
2 tablespoons canola oil
2 egg whites, beaten
½ cup whole wheat flour
2 tablespoons turbino
¼ teaspoon salt
1 teaspoon baking powder
⅓ cup raisins
1 cup mixed berries (raspberry, blueberry, blackberry, or strawberry)

1. In a bowl, combine milk and oats. Let stand 5 minutes.

2. Add oil and beaten egg whites and mix well. Add flour, 1 tablespoon of turbino, salt, and baking powder and stir just until dry ingredients are moist.

PER SERVING
Calories 108
Calories from Fat 30
Percent Total Calories From:
Fat 28%
Protein 14%
Carbohydrates 58%
Percent RDA:
Vitamin A 1%
Vitamin C 1%
Calcium 0%
Iron 3%

Nutrient	Amount per Serving	% Daily Value
Total Fat	3 g	5%
Saturated Fat	0 g	2%
Cholesterol	0 mg	0%
Sodium	119 mg	5%
Total Carbohydrate	16 g	5%
Dietary Fiber	1 g	4%
Sugars	0 g	
Protein	4 g	

3. Drop ¼ cup batter at a time on a hot, lightly oiled griddle. Turn when top is bubbly and sides are brown and cook on other side until done.

4. Combine raisins, berries, and remaining turbino. Top pancakes with fruit mixture and serve.

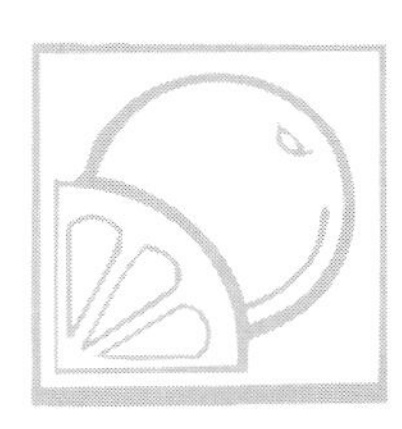

Broiled Grapefruit

2 SERVINGS

1 grapefruit, cut in half
2 tablespoons turbino
½ cup plain nonfat yogurt
1 kiwi, peeled and sliced
½ papaya, peeled and sliced
4 mint leaves, chopped

1. Preheat broiler.

2. Sprinkle turbino on grapefruit. Place on broiler pan and broil for 3 minutes.

3. In a bowl, mix together the kiwi, papaya, and yogurt.

4. Serve grapefruit topped with spoonfuls of yogurt/fruit mixture. Garnish with chopped mint.

PER SERVING
Calories 145
Calories from Fat 23
Percent Total Calories From:
Fat 16%
Protein 11%
Carbohydrates 73%
Percent RDA:
Vitamin A 14%
Vitamin C 22%
Calcium 0%
Iron 7%

Nutrient	Amount per Serving	% Daily Value
Total Fat	3 g	4%
Saturated Fat	1 g	7%
Cholesterol	8 mg	3%
Sodium	35 mg	1%
Total Carbohydrate	27 g	9%
Dietary Fiber	1 g	5%
Sugars	0 g	
Protein	4 g	

Egg White French Toast

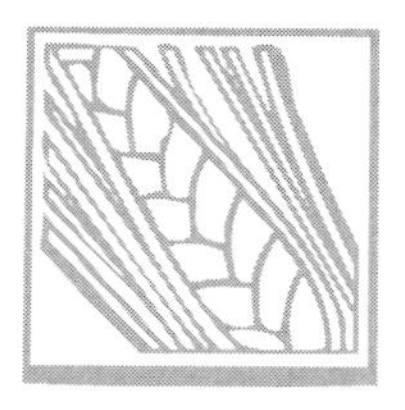

2 SERVINGS

3 egg whites, beaten
1 teaspoon ground cinnamon
1 teaspoon turbino
Pinch nutmeg
4 slices bread, whole wheat or oat bran
1 tablespoon canola oil
1 cup sliced or chopped fresh fruit
1 teaspoon chopped mint

1. In a bowl, mix eggs, cinnamon, turbino, and nutmeg.
2. Saturate bread with egg mixture.
3. Heat the canola oil in a sauté pan on medium heat, and cook bread until brown on each side.
4. Arrange 1 slice of bread on a plate, cover with fruit, then top with the second slice of bread and top with mint.

PER SERVING
Calories 296
Calories from Fat 83
Percent Total Calories From:
Fat 28%
Protein 14%
Carbohydrates 58%
Percent RDA:
Vitamin A 1%
Vitamin C 7%
Calcium 0%
Iron 14%

Nutrient	Amount per Serving	% Daily Value
Total Fat	9 g	14%
Saturated Fat	1 g	6%
Cholesterol	2 mg	1%
Sodium	373 mg	16%
Total Carbohydrate	43 g	14%
Dietary Fiber	2 g	7%
Sugars	0 g	
Protein	10 g	

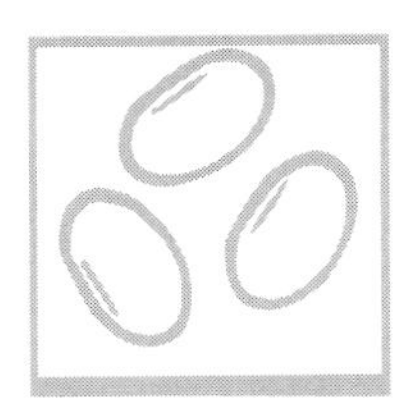

Egg White Frittata with Salsa

4 SERVINGS

Salsa

¼ onion, diced
1 green onion, sliced
2 plum tomatoes, diced
2 tablespoons chopped fresh cilantro
Juice of 1 lime

Frittata

5 egg whites, beaten
Pinch pepper
1 teaspoon olive oil
¼ onion, sliced
1 clove garlic, minced

1. In a bowl, mix all salsa ingredients. Refrigerate 20 minutes while you make the fritatta.

2. Preheat oven to 350 degrees F.

3. In a mixing bowl, combine egg whites and pepper and beat well.

PER SERVING
Calories 52
Calories from Fat 13
Percent Total Calories From:
Fat 24%
Protein 38%
Carbohydrates 38%
Percent RDA:
Vitamin A 0%
Vitamin C 11%
Calcium 0%
Iron 2%

Nutrient	Amount per Serving	% Daily Value
Total Fat	1 g	2%
Saturated Fat	0 g	1%
Cholesterol	0 mg	0%
Sodium	70 mg	3%
Total Carbohydrate	5 g	2%
Dietary Fiber	0 g	1%
Sugars	0 g	
Protein	5 g	

4. Heat olive oil in a nonstick ovenproof omelet pan. Add onion slices and cook on medium until golden in color, shaking pan to ensure that the onions are cooked evenly. Add garlic to onion slices; stir.

5. Drizzle egg whites into pan while swirling pan, and place pan in preheated oven. Bake 4 to 5 minutes, or until egg frittata is set.

6. Loosen frittata from omelet pan by running a rubber spatula around the outside of the frittata. Place a large, round plate over omelet pan and invert the omelet pan and plate quickly, letting the frittata fall onto the plate.

7. Garnish with salsa and serve.

Rice with Fruit

10 SERVINGS

- 2 cups soy milk
- 2 cups water
- ¼ cup turbino
- ⅛ teaspoon ground cloves
- ¾ teaspoon nutmeg
- 1⅓ cups brown rice, uncooked
- 1 mango, chopped
- ½ pineapple, chopped
- 1 peach, chopped
- 2 tablespoons crushed walnuts

1. In a saucepan, mix soy milk, water, turbino, cloves, and nutmeg. Bring to a boil.

2. Add rice, reduce heat, cover, and let simmer until rice is cooked.

3. Mix in fresh fruit and top with walnuts. Serve.

PER SERVING
Calories 189
Calories from Fat 23
Percent Total Calories From:
Fat 12%
Protein 8%
Carbohydrates 80%
Percent RDA:
Vitamin A 18%
Vitamin C 34%
Calcium 0%
Iron 10%

Nutrient	Amount per Serving	% Daily Value
Total Fat	3 g	4%
Saturated Fat	0 g	2%
Cholesterol	0 mg	0%
Sodium	8 mg	0%
Total Carbohydrate	38 g	13%
Dietary Fiber	1 g	4%
Sugars	0 g	
Protein	4 g	

Blueberry-Banana Muffins

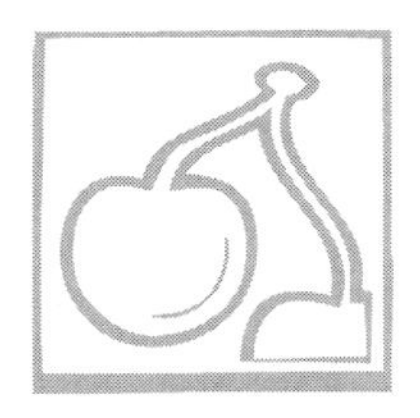

10 SERVINGS

½ cup whole wheat flour
1½ cups rolled oats
2 teaspoons baking powder
½ teaspoon baking soda
2 tablespoons turbino
2 pinches nutmeg
1 cup blueberries
½ banana, sliced
¼ cup molasses
¼ cup apples, pureed
½ cup soy milk
2 egg whites

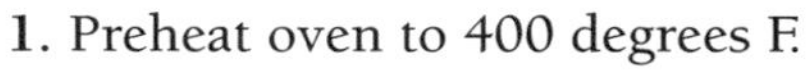

1. Preheat oven to 400 degrees F.
2. In large bowl, mix flour, oats, baking powder, baking soda, turbino, and nutmeg. Stir in blueberries, bananas, molasses, and apples. Add soy milk and egg whites and mix gently.
3. Line a muffin tin with foil muffin cups. Fill cups two-thirds full and bake for 25 minutes, or until a toothpick inserted in the center comes out clean.

PER SERVING
Calories 93
Calories from Fat 11
Percent Total Calories From:
Fat 12%
Protein 14%
Carbohydrates 74%
Percent RDA:
Vitamin A 1%
Vitamin C 4%
Calcium 0%
Iron 11%

Nutrient	Amount per Serving	% Daily Value
Total Fat	1 g	2%
Saturated Fat	0 g	1%
Cholesterol	0 mg	0%
Sodium	133 mg	6%
Total Carbohydrate	17 g	6%
Dietary Fiber	2 g	6%
Sugars	0 g	
Protein	3 g	

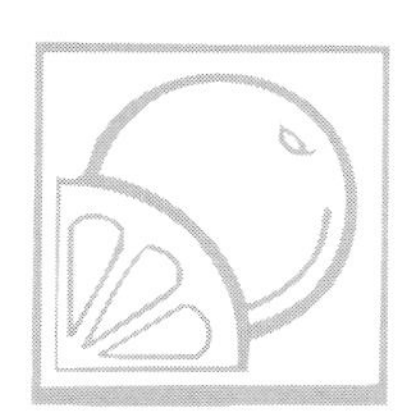

Baked Banana with Granola and Mango

8 SERVINGS

Granola

3 cups raw wheat germ
2 cups rolled oats
1 cup wheat bran
½ cup soy flour
¼ cup canola oil
¼ cup turbino
1 vanilla bean
1 cup sunflower seeds, toasted
1 cup pumpkin seeds, toasted
1 cup raisins

Fruit

4 bananas, sliced lengthwise
2 mangos, sliced

PER SERVING
Calories 544
Calories from Fat 222
Percent Total Calories From:
Fat 41%
Protein 15%
Carbohydrates 44%
Percent RDA:
Vitamin A 2%
Vitamin C 9%
Calcium 0%
Iron 33%

Nutrient	Amount per Serving	% Daily Value
Total Fat	25 g	38%
Saturated Fat	3 g	15%
Cholesterol	0 mg	0%
Sodium	9 mg	0%
Total Carbohydrate	60 g	20%
Dietary Fiber	7 g	29%
Sugars	0 g	
Protein	21 g	

1. Preheat oven to 350 degrees F.

2. In a bowl, mix all granola ingredients except seeds and raisins.

3. Spread in a shallow baking dish and bake for 45 minutes, stirring twice.

4. Store granola and the vanilla bean in an airtight container.

5. Put bananas in a shallow baking dish and bake at 350 degrees F. for 10 minutes.

6. Put bananas on a plate and serve with sliced fresh mango and granola mixture. Top with toasted seeds and raisins.

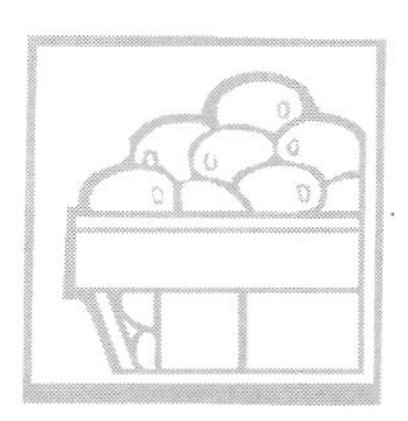

Rice Water

10 SERVINGS

1 cup white rice, cooked
2 cups water
4 tablespoons vanilla nonfat yogurt
1 teaspoon ground cinnamon
Pinch nutmeg
Honey, to taste

1. Soak rice in water overnight.
2. In a blender or food processor, combine soaked rice, and the remainder of the water, yogurt, cinnamon, and nutmeg and puree.
3. Chill mixture, and sweeten with honey. The mixture should be about the consistency of cooked oatmeal. Add more water if too thick.

PER SERVING
Calories 81
Calories from Fat 4
Percent Total Calories From:
Fat 5%
Protein 8%
Carbohydrates 88%
Percent RDA:
Vitamin A 0%
Vitamin C 0%
Calcium 0%
Iron 6%

Nutrient	Amount per Serving	% Daily Value
Total Fat	0 g	1%
Saturated Fat	0 g	1%
Cholesterol	1 mg	0%
Sodium	3 mg	0%
Total Carbohydrate	18 g	6%
Dietary Fiber	0 g	1%
Sugars	0 g	
Protein	2 g	

Chilled Fresh Fruit Breakfast Soup

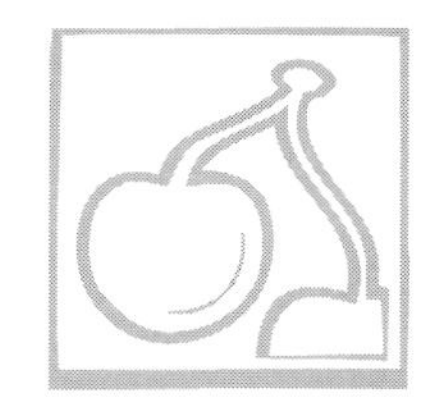

6 SERVINGS

½ cup fresh apricots, pitted and sliced
½ cup fresh peaches, pitted, peeled, and sliced
½ cup tart cherries, pitted
1 vanilla bean, split
1 cinnamon stick
2 tablespoons lemon juice
Pinch turbino
¼ cup plain nonfat yogurt
½ cup Granola (see recipe, page 36)

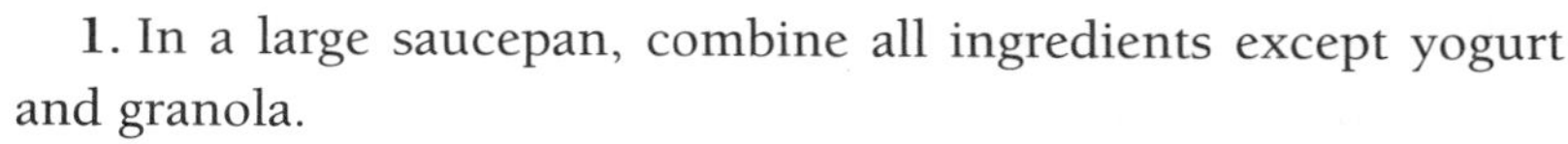

1. In a large saucepan, combine all ingredients except yogurt and granola.

2. Add 6 cups of water, bring to a boil, reduce heat, and simmer for approximately 15 minutes. Let cool.

3. Remove cinnamon stick and vanilla bean, put mixture in blender, and puree.

4. Pour into bowls; swirl in yogurt and garnish with granola. Serve.

PER SERVING
Calories 83
Calories from Fat 29
Percent Total Calories From:
- Fat 35%
- Protein 10%
- Carbohydrates 55%

Percent RDA:
- Vitamin A 8%
- Vitamin C 9%
- Calcium 0%
- Iron 3%

Nutrient	Amount per Serving	% Daily Value
Total Fat	3 g	5%
Saturated Fat	1 g	4%
Cholesterol	1 mg	0%
Sodium	6 mg	0%
Total Carbohydrate	11 g	4%
Dietary Fiber	0 g	2%
Sugars	0 g	
Protein	2 g	

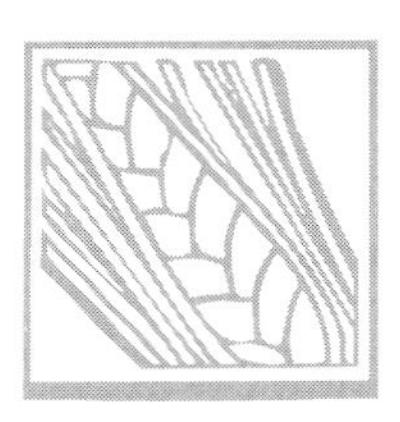

Stacked Waffles

12 SERVINGS

1 apple, peeled, cored, and sliced
½ cup pitted prunes
1 cinnamon stick
3 tablespoons turbino
3 tablespoons water
3 cups waffle mix, organic preferred
2 tablespoons mixed dried fruit
3 tablespoons plain nonfat yogurt

1. In a small pan, combine apples, prunes, cinnamon and turbino. Add water and simmer for 20 minutes.

2. Cook waffles according to directions on box. Place fruit mixture on top of waffle and cover with second waffle. Top with fruit and yogurt mixture.

PER SERVING
Calories 36
Calories from Fat 2
Percent Total Calories From:
Fat 6%
Protein 4%
Carbohydrates 90%
Percent RDA:
Vitamin A 4%
Vitamin C 2%
Calcium 0%
Iron 2%

Nutrient	Amount per Serving	% Daily Value
Total Fat	0 g	0%
Saturated Fat	0 g	0%
Cholesterol	0 mg	0%
Sodium	2 mg	0%
Total Carbohydrate	8 g	3%
Dietary Fiber	1 g	2%
Sugars	0 g	
Protein	0 g	

Baked Apples

6 SERVINGS

¼ cup fresh cranberries, cooked
1 tablespoon fresh blueberries
2 tablespoons Granola (see recipe, page 36)
2 apples, cored, tops cut off
2 tablespoons plain nonfat yogurt
2 mint leaves, garnish

1. Preheat oven to 350 degrees F.
2. Mix cranberries, blueberries, and granola in a bowl.
3. Fill apples with fruit mixture and place apples on a baking tray. Bake until apples are soft.
4. Top apples with yogurt and garnish with mint.

PER SERVING
Calories 64
Calories from Fat 10
Percent Total Calories From:
- Fat 16%
- Protein 4%
- Carbohydrates 80%

Percent RDA:
- Vitamin A 1%
- Vitamin C 8%
- Calcium 0%
- Iron 2%

Nutrient	Amount per Serving	% Daily Value
Total Fat	1 g	2%
Saturated Fat	0 g	1%
Cholesterol	1 mg	0%
Sodium	3 mg	0%
Total Carbohydrate	13 g	4%
Dietary Fiber	1 g	6%
Sugars	0 g	
Protein	1 g	

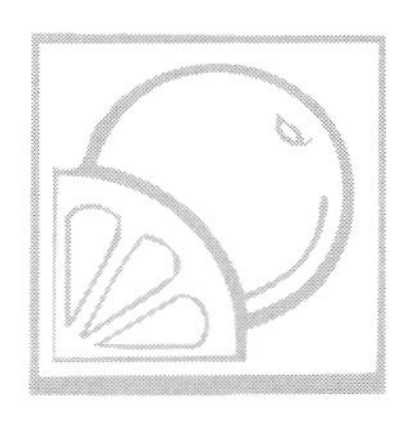

Cold Cantaloupe

4 SERVINGS

1 cantaloupe
½ cup plain nonfat yogurt
4 mint leaves, chopped
Pinch nutmeg
Juice of ½ lemon
Pinch turbino
1 cup strawberries

1. Cut cantaloupe in half, remove seeds, and carefully scoop flesh from melon, reserving the shells.
2. In a blender, puree cantaloupe, yogurt, mint, nutmeg, lemon juice, and turbino.
2. Pour pureed mixture into melon shell. Chill.
3. Garnish with strawberries and serve.

PER SERVING
Calories 94
Calories from Fat 16
Percent Total Calories From:
Fat 18%
Protein 11%
Carbohydrates 71%
Percent RDA:
Vitamin A 88%
Vitamin C 138%
Calcium 0%
Iron 5%

Nutrient	Amount per Serving	% Daily Value
Total Fat	2 g	3%
Saturated Fat	1 g	4%
Cholesterol	4 mg	1%
Sodium	28 mg	1%
Total Carbohydrate	17 g	6%
Dietary Fiber	1 g	3%
Sugars	0 g	
Protein	3 g	

Smoked Salmon with Scrambled Eggs

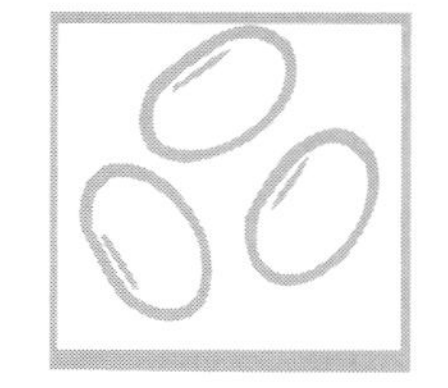

4 SERVINGS

3 ounces fresh spinach, chopped
1 tablespoon freshly squeezed lemon juice
2 tablespoons olive oil
6 ounces smoked salmon, crumbled
1 green onion, sliced
1 sprig fresh thyme
3 egg whites, beaten
Pinch salt
Pinch pepper

1. In a medium skillet, combine spinach, lemon juice, and a few drops of water. Cook over medium heat until wilted. Put in a bowl and set aside.

2. Wipe skillet clean, and heat olive oil over medium heat. Add salmon, green onion, and thyme and cook, stirring.

3. Add egg whites, season with salt and pepper, and stir constantly until cooked. Serve over spinach.

PER SERVING
Calories 134
Calories from Fat 88
Percent Total Calories From:
Fat 66%
Protein 29%
Carbohydrates 5%
Percent RDA:
Vitamin A 29%
Vitamin C 13%
Calcium 0%
Iron 8%

Nutrient	Amount per Serving	% Daily Value
Total Fat	10 g	15%
Saturated Fat	2 g	8%
Cholesterol	18 mg	6%
Sodium	817 mg	34%
Total Carbohydrate	2 g	1%
Dietary Fiber	0 g	1%
Sugars	0 g	
Protein	10 g	

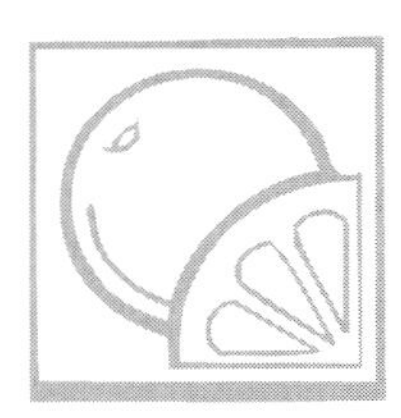

8 SERVINGS

Blintzes

Blintzes

5 tablespoons soy milk, chilled
5 tablespoons water, chilled
2 egg whites, beaten
⅓ cup white or wheat flour
Pinch salt

Filling

1 cup low-fat cottage cheese
2 tablespoons raisins
Dash ground cinnamon
1 tablespoon turbino
½ orange, sliced
Juice of ½ orange

PER SERVING
Calories 69
Calories from Fat 13
Percent Total Calories From:
Fat 19%
Protein 30%
Carbohydrates 51%
Percent RDA:
Vitamin A 2%
Vitamin C 15%
Calcium 0%
Iron 1%

Nutrient	Amount per Serving	% Daily Value
Total Fat	1 g	2%
Saturated Fat	1 g	4%
Cholesterol	4 mg	1%
Sodium	412 mg	17%
Total Carbohydrate	9 g	3%
Dietary Fiber	0 g	1%
Sugars	0 g	
Protein	5 g	

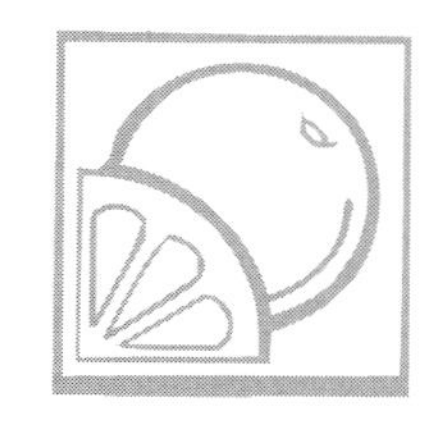

1. In a bowl, mix blintz ingredients. Cover and refrigerate for 1 hour.

2. In another bowl, combine filling ingredients.

3. Heat a nonstick skillet, and spoon in just enough batter to fill bottom of pan. Cook blintz 45 seconds, flip it over, and cook 45 seconds on the other side. Stack blintzes on waxed paper until done.

4. Place a spoonful of cheese/fruit mixture into each cooked blintz. Tuck in ends and roll up.

5. Sprinkle blintzes with fresh lemon juice and turbino, if desired, and serve.

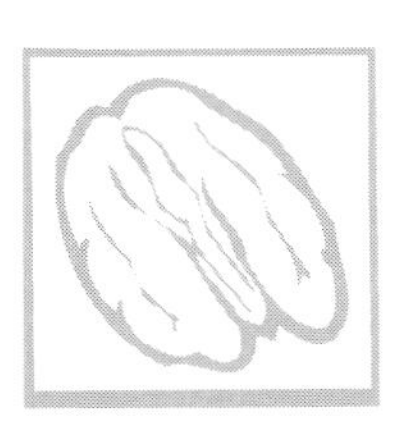

ADA

10 SERVINGS

ADA Pancakes

2 cups cracked wheat
1 cup brown rice flour
3 cups water
½ teaspoon salt
½ cup fresh cilantro leaves, finely chopped
3 green onions, minced

Topping

1 cup organic apple juice
1 peach, pitted and sliced
2 tablespoons raisins
2 tablespoons white vinegar
2 tablespoons turbino
1 teaspoon ground cinnamon
2 pinches ground cloves
2 pinches ground cardamom

PER SERVING
Calories 184
Calories from Fat 8
Percent Total Calories From:
Fat 4%
Protein 10%
Carbohydrates 85%
Percent RDA:
Vitamin A 1%
Vitamin C 19%
Calcium 0%
Iron 7%

Nutrient	Amount per Serving	% Daily Value
Total Fat	1 g	1%
Saturated Fat	0 g	1%
Cholesterol	0 mg	0%
Sodium	124 mg	5%
Total Carbohydrate	39 g	13%
Dietary Fiber	1 g	4%
Sugars	0 g	
Protein	5 g	

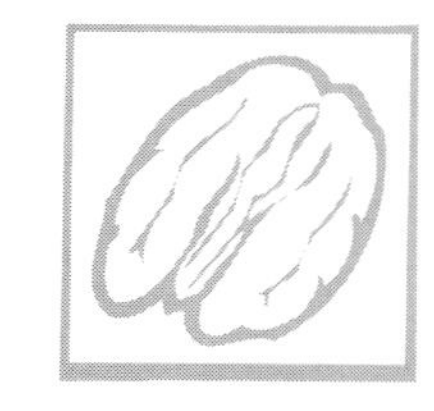

1. Grind cracked wheat in blender until it becomes fine meal.

2. In a medium bowl, combine rice flour, cracked wheat, water, and salt. Let stand overnight.

3. Make the topping: Combine all ingredients in saucepan and bring to boil. Simmer on low for 30 minutes.

4. To make pancakes, mix cilantro and minced onions into cracked wheat mixture.

5. Heat a nonstick griddle. Spoon batter onto griddle and cook for a few minutes on each side.

6. Spoon topping over ADA and serve.

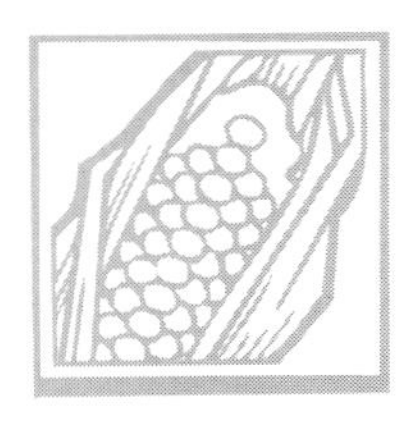

Breakfast Mix

6 SERVINGS

¼ cup pumpkin seeds, shelled
¼ cup sunflower seeds, shelled
¼ cup mixed nuts, unsalted
1 apple, cored, peeled, and chopped
1 banana, sliced
4 tablespoons honey

1. Mix all ingredients together.
2. Serve with milk or yogurt like granola.

PER SERVING
Calories 137
Calories from Fat 36
Percent Total Calories From:
Fat 26%
Protein 6%
Carbohydrates 68%
Percent RDA:
Vitamin A 1%
Vitamin C 6%
Calcium 0%
Iron 4%

Nutrient	Amount per Serving	% Daily Value
Total Fat	4 g	6%
Saturated Fat	0 g	2%
Cholesterol	0 mg	0%
Sodium	2 mg	0%
Total Carbohydrate	23 g	8%
Dietary Fiber	2 g	7%
Sugars	0 g	
Protein	2 g	

Fried Polenta with Mixed Berries

8 SERVINGS

1 cup cornmeal
1 cup cold water
2 ounces low-fat cottage cheese
¼ cup plain yogurt
1 teaspoon canola oil
8 raspberries
8 boysenberries
10 blackberries
20 blueberries
6 strawberries

1. In a saucepan, whisk cornmeal and water together and cook over medium heat, stirring with a wooden spoon, until thickened.

2. In a bowl, blend cottage cheese and yogurt.

3. Pour cornmeal onto a cutting board and cut into squares. Top each square with a spoonful of cheese and yogurt mixture.

4. Heat oil in nonstick skillet over medium heat. Place cornmeal squares in pan and fry until crisp. Garnish with any amount of fresh berries and serve.

PER SERVING
Calories 86
Calories from Fat 13
Percent Total Calories From:
Fat 15%
Protein 13%
Carbohydrates 72%
Percent RDA:
Vitamin A 2%
Vitamin C 13%
Calcium 0%
Iron 2%

Nutrient	Amount per Serving	% Daily Value
Total Fat	1 g	2%
Saturated Fat	0 g	2%
Cholesterol	2 mg	1%
Sodium	33 mg	1%
Total Carbohydrate	16 g	5%
Dietary Fiber	0 g	1%
Sugars	0 g	
Protein	3 g	

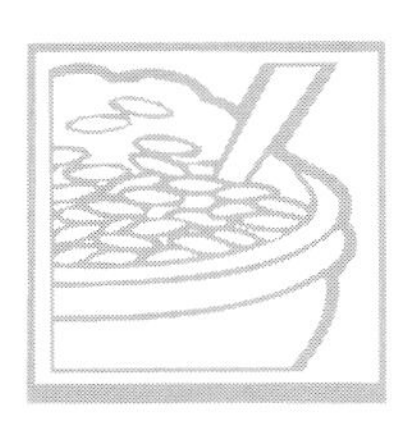

Indian Breakfast

10 SERVINGS

Curry Powder

2 teaspoons coriander seeds
½ teaspoon cumin seeds
2 teaspoons ground cardamom
2 cloves
½ teaspoon mace
⅛ teaspoon allspice
1 bay leaf, cut up
3 sprigs fresh thyme
1 teaspoon fenugreek
2 teaspoons turmeric

Rice Mixture

1 tablespoon olive oil
2 cups chopped onions
1½ tablespoons curry powder
¾ cup split peas, cooked
½ cup white or brown cooked rice

PER SERVING
Calories 105
Calories from Fat 20
Percent Total Calories From:
Fat 19%
Protein 18%
Carbohydrates 63%
Percent RDA:
Vitamin A 1%
Vitamin C 5%
Calcium 0%
Iron 12%

Nutrient	Amount per Serving	% Daily Value
Total Fat	2 g	3%
Saturated Fat	0 g	1%
Cholesterol	0 mg	0%
Sodium	5 mg	0%
Total Carbohydrate	17 g	6%
Dietary Fiber	1 g	5%
Sugars	0 g	
Protein	5 g	

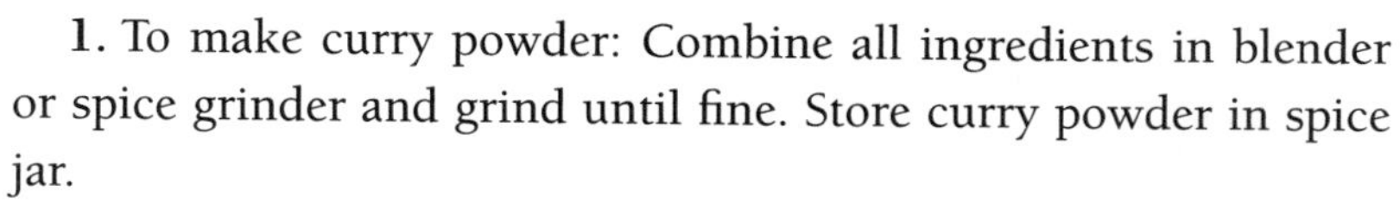

1. To make curry powder: Combine all ingredients in blender or spice grinder and grind until fine. Store curry powder in spice jar.

2. Heat olive oil in large skillet and cook onions until transparent.

3. Add curry powder and mix well. Add peas, stir, and serve over rice.

Consommé with Lemon and Angel Hair

2 SERVINGS

2 cups beef consommé
1 ounce angel hair pasta, uncooked
½ lemon, sliced

1. In a saucepan, bring consommé to boil and add pasta. Simmer until pasta is done.

2. Serve with sliced lemon for a hot, morning broth.

PER SERVING
Calories 67
Calories from Fat 11
Percent Total Calories From:
Fat 17%
Protein 29%
Carbohydrates 54%
Percent RDA:
Vitamin A 0%
Vitamin C 13%
Calcium 0%
Iron 3%

Nutrient	Amount per Serving	% Daily Value
Total Fat	1 g	2%
Saturated Fat	0 g	2%
Cholesterol	12 mg	4%
Sodium	789 mg	33%
Total Carbohydrate	9 g	3%
Dietary Fiber	0 g	0%
Sugars	0 g	
Protein	5 g	

Poor Man's Pudding

2 SERVINGS

2 slices whole wheat bread, cubed
1 apple, cored and diced
1 cup soy milk
1 egg white
1 tablespoon raisins
1 teaspoon turbino
1 teaspoon vanilla extract
¼ teaspoon ground cinnamon
Dash nutmeg
3 strawberries, sliced
2 mint leaves, chopped

1. Preheat oven to 350 degrees F.
2. In a small bowl, mix all ingredients except strawberries and mint.
3. Pour into an ovenproof nonstick pan and bake for 35 to 40 minutes.
4. Garnish servings with strawberries and mint and serve.

PER SERVING
Calories 224
Calories from Fat 34
Percent Total Calories From:
Fat 15%
Protein 15%
Carbohydrates 70%
Percent RDA:
Vitamin A 3%
Vitamin C 37%
Calcium 0%
Iron 16%

Nutrient	Amount per Serving	% Daily Value
Total Fat	4 g	6%
Saturated Fat	1 g	3%
Cholesterol	1 mg	0%
Sodium	191 mg	8%
Total Carbohydrate	39 g	13%
Dietary Fiber	3 g	12%
Sugars	0 g	
Protein	8 g	

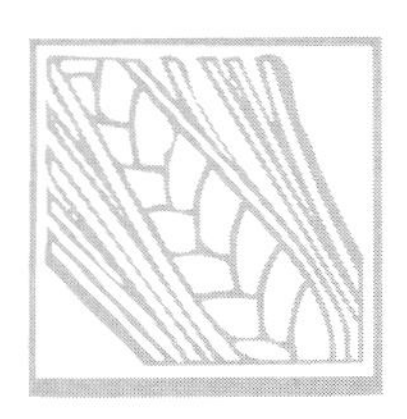

Multigrain Prune Muffins

10 SERVINGS

¾ cup flour
½ cup whole wheat flour
½ cup oats
⅓ cup turbino
¼ cup cornmeal
¼ cup wheat germ
1½ teaspoons baking soda
¼ teaspoon salt
1 cup pitted prunes, chopped
1 cup plain nonfat yogurt
1 tablespoon flaxseed oil
1 egg white
1 teaspoon orange zest
Fresh berries for garnish

PER SERVING
Calories 153
Calories from Fat 15
Percent Total Calories From:
- Fat 10%
- Protein 13%
- Carbohydrates 77%

Percent RDA:
- Vitamin A 7%
- Vitamin C 1%
- Calcium 0%
- Iron 6%

Nutrient	Amount per Serving	% Daily Value
Total Fat	2 g	3%
Saturated Fat	1 g	3%
Cholesterol	3 mg	1%
Sodium	200 mg	8%
Total Carbohydrate	30 g	10%
Dietary Fiber	1 g	2%
Sugars	0 g	
Protein	5 g	

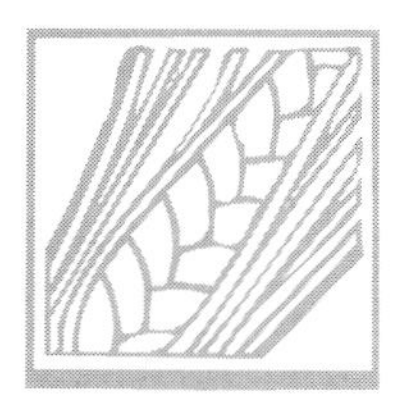

4 SERVINGS

1. Preheat oven to 400 degrees F.

2. In a large bowl, combine flours, oats, turbino, cornmeal, wheat germ, baking soda, and salt.

3. In a small bowl, combine prunes, yogurt, flaxseed oil, egg white, and orange zest. Stir well to mix.

4. Make a well in center of the flour and oat mixture. Add prune mixture to dry ingredients, stirring until just moistened.

5. Pour batter into greased muffin pans and bake for 20 minutes. Serve with fresh berries.

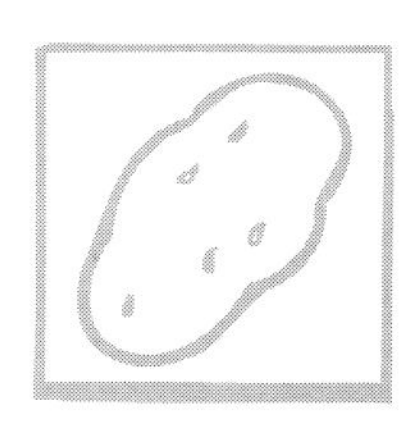

Far East Omelet

2 SERVINGS

2 teaspoons sesame oil
½ carrot, peeled and grated
1 teaspoon chopped garlic
1 teaspoon peeled and chopped fresh ginger
¼ cup bean sprouts
4 egg whites, beaten
¼ cup green onions, chopped

1. Heat sesame oil in a medium nonstick skillet over medium heat.

2. Add carrot, garlic, ginger, and bean sprouts and sauté for 1 minute.

3. Add egg whites and let set about 1 minute. Sprinkle green onion over top.

4. Fold omelet in half and slide onto a plate.

5. Serve with green tea.

PER SERVING
Calories 94
Calories from Fat 41
Percent Total Calories From:
Fat 44%
Protein 34%
Carbohydrates 22%
Percent RDA:
Vitamin A 102%
Vitamin C 11%
Calcium 0%
Iron 3%

Nutrient	Amount per Serving	% Daily Value
Total Fat	5 g	7%
Saturated Fat	1 g	3%
Cholesterol	0 mg	0%
Sodium	119 mg	5%
Total Carbohydrate	5 g	2%
Dietary Fiber	0 g	2%
Sugars	0 g	
Protein	8 g	

Turkey Sausage Patty

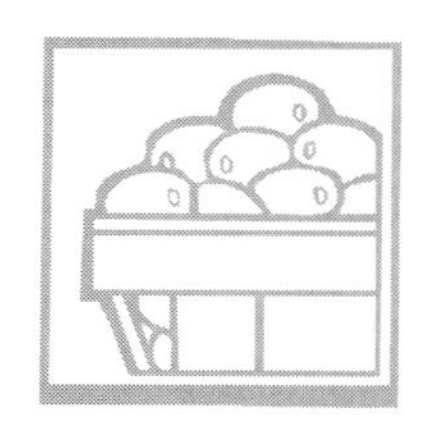

8 SERVINGS

1 pound ground turkey
1½ teaspoons salt
1½ teaspoons pepper
1 teaspoon dried sage
¾ teaspoon ground ginger
¾ teaspoon allspice
¼ teaspoon red pepper

1. In a medium bowl, mix all ingredients.
2. Shape into patties, place on a heated nonstick skillet, and cook until well done.
3. Serve alone or with egg dishes.

PER SERVING
Calories 82
Calories from Fat 38
Percent Total Calories From:
Fat 47%
Protein 50%
Carbohydrates 3%
Percent RDA:
Vitamin A 0%
Vitamin C 0%
Calcium 0%
Iron 4%

Nutrient	Amount per Serving	% Daily Value
Total Fat	4 g	6%
Saturated Fat	1 g	6%
Cholesterol	41 mg	14%
Sodium	486 mg	20%
Total Carbohydrate	1 g	0%
Dietary Fiber	0 g	0%
Sugars	0 g	
Protein	10 g	

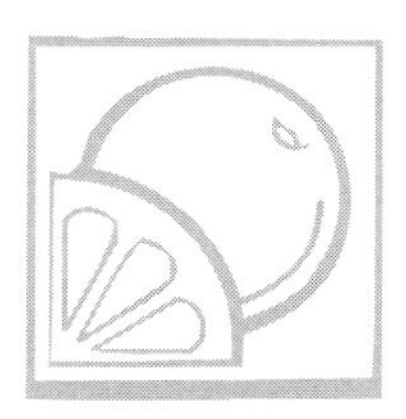

Breakfast Salad

6 SERVINGS

1 cup mixed salad greens
⅓ cup nonfat cottage cheese
¼ cup alfalfa sprouts
1 teaspoon sunflower seeds
½ blood orange, peeled and sectioned
½ orange, peeled and sectioned
⅓ cup canned mandarin orange sections
½ banana, peeled and sliced

1. Place the salad greens on a plate and top with a scoop of cottage cheese. Sprinkle with alfalfa sprouts and seeds.

2. Garnish with oranges and banana and serve.

PER SERVING
Calories 49
Calories from Fat 9
Percent Total Calories From:
- Fat 18%
- Protein 18%
- Carbohydrates 65%

Percent RDA:
- Vitamin A 18%
- Vitamin C 34%
- Calcium 0%
- Iron 2%

Nutrient	Amount per Serving	% Daily Value
Total Fat	1 g	1%
Saturated Fat	0 g	2%
Cholesterol	2 mg	1%
Sodium	51 mg	2%
Total Carbohydrate	8 g	3%
Dietary Fiber	0 g	1%
Sugars	0 g	
Protein	2 g	

Breakfast Leeks

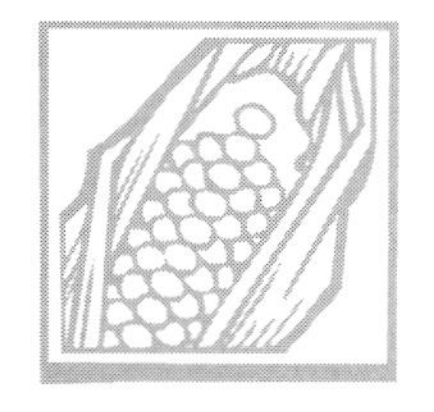

2 SERVINGS

1 tablespoon olive oil
1 leek, washed and diced
2 egg whites
1 teaspoon chopped fresh parsley
1 teaspoon chopped fresh basil
1 teaspoon fresh thyme
Dash salt and pepper

1. Heat oil in nonstick pan over medium heat. Add leek, stir, and cook for 2 minutes.

2. Add eggs, herbs, salt, and pepper, and stir. Cook until bottom of eggs are set. Flip over, cook 1 more minute. Serve.

PER SERVING
Calories 129
Calories from Fat 72
Percent Total Calories From:
Fat 56%
Protein 14%
Carbohydrates 30%
Percent RDA:
Vitamin A 3%
Vitamin C 13%
Calcium 0%
Iron 14%

Nutrient	Amount per Serving	% Daily Value
Total Fat	8 g	12%
Saturated Fat	1 g	5%
Cholesterol	0 mg	0%
Sodium	69 mg	3%
Total Carbohydrate	10 g	3%
Dietary Fiber	1 g	4%
Sugars	0 g	
Protein	5 g	

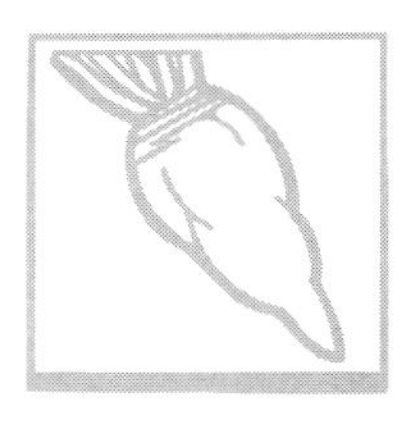

Spicy Johnny Cakes

10 SERVINGS

1 cup yellow cornmeal
¾ cup wheat flour
2 tablespoons turbino
2 teaspoons baking powder
¼ teaspoon chili powder
Pinch salt
Pinch pepper
2 tablespoons canola oil
¾ cup soy milk
1 egg white
1 tablespoon chopped canned chili chipotle adobados (mild)
2 tablespoons frozen corn kernels

1. Preheat oven to 400 degrees F.

2. In a medium bowl, combine cornmeal, flour, turbino, baking powder, chili powder, salt, and pepper. Mix in remaining ingredients and stir well.

3. Pour batter into an ovenproof nonstick skillet and bake for 20 minutes. Serve with egg dishes.

PER SERVING
Calories 120
Calories from Fat 31
Percent Total Calories From:
Fat 26%
Protein 10%
Carbohydrates 64%
Percent RDA:
Vitamin A 6%
Vitamin C 2%
Calcium 0%
Iron 3%

Nutrient	Amount per Serving	% Daily Value
Total Fat	3 g	5%
Saturated Fat	0 g	1%
Cholesterol	0 mg	0%
Sodium	331 mg	14%
Total Carbohydrate	19 g	6%
Dietary Fiber	0 g	1%
Sugars	0 g	
Protein	3 g	

Natural Breakfast Cereal

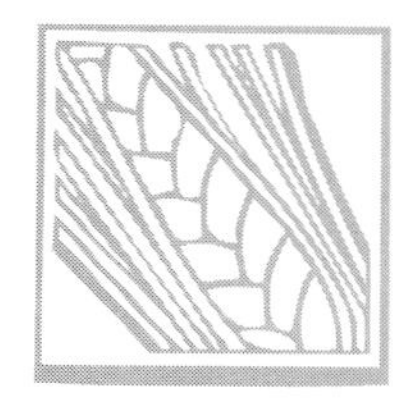

⅔ cup wheat berries
⅓ cup whole oats
1 tablespoon sunflower seeds
½ teaspoon honey

6 SERVINGS

1. Rinse wheat, oats, and sunflower seeds.

2. In a saucepan, combine all ingredients with 2½ cups cold water. Bring to a boil, reduce heat, cover, and steam for 3 hours.

3. Serve with wheat germ and honey to taste.

PER SERVING
Calories 88
Calories from Fat 12
Percent Total Calories From:
Fat 14%
Protein 15%
Carbohydrates 72%
Percent RDA:
Vitamin A 0%
Vitamin C 0%
Calcium 0%
Iron 5%

Nutrient	Amount per Serving	% Daily Value
Total Fat	1 g	2%
Saturated Fat	0 g	1%
Cholesterol	0 mg	0%
Sodium	0 mg	0%
Total Carbohydrate	16 g	5%
Dietary Fiber	1 g	2%
Sugars	0 g	
Protein	3 g	

Chapter 4

LUNCH

Powering Your Way Through the Day

WELL, YOU'VE MADE IT THIS FAR! YOU'VE STARTED YOUR day off on the right foot, with a wholesome and healthful meal. But, like everything else, the real world intrudes. The boss calls you, you've got a project that's due, you're beginning to drag, yet that forty-five to sixty-minute lunch time certainly seems like it could be an enticing block of time to do something else. Maybe you should skip lunch and get that last bit of work done, or run that last errand, or drop off your child's project to school. Don't do it!

You must recognize that every single meal that you take into your body serves as precious fuel or medication and is so very important. Choose the right fuel, and you can power yourself ahead for a fulfilling and satisfying start to the next phase of your day's journey.

This is very important, because as you know, the afternoon looms ahead and you need energy. No, we're not talking about the power bar or candy bar type of energy that we all think of. You don't need a quick burst, but rather a sustained, maintained power drive to get you through the afternoon. You need food that will help you on your way home and keep you thinking positively. And what's more important, you don't want to have an impulse to reach for a quick fix candy bar or bag of potato chips, only to find out that this drains your energy resources for later, leaving you even lower than you are right now. No, you can't cheat yourself. Lunch is too important.

In this chapter we discuss many wholesome and nutritious meals that are not only good for you, they are also tasty and delicious. Many of them can be prepared in a short time, leaving you time to do all the other things that you didn't think you'd have time for. But most of all, a good lunch will provide you with the energy, strength, stamina, and fortitude to move forward. Each day is a marathon, and each minute is important. That's why you must recognize that every single meal that you take into your body serves as precious fuel or medication and is so very important. Choose the right fuel, and you can power yourself ahead for a fulfilling and satisfying start to the next phase of your day's journey.

Tuna Couscous Salad

4 SERVINGS

Salad

1 6-ounce tuna fillet
Pinch salt
Pinch pepper
1 cup couscous, cooked

Dressing

2 cucumbers, peeled and seeded
Salt and pepper, to taste
1 clove garlic
1 teaspoon chopped fresh dill
½ cup plain nonfat yogurt

1. Preheat oven to 350 degrees F.
2. Salt and pepper tuna and bake until medium doneness, approximately 8 minutes.
3. In a blender, puree all dressing ingredients.
4. Toss couscous with dressing, flake tuna on salad mixture, and serve.

PER SERVING
Calories 242
Calories from Fat 22
Percent Total Calories From:
Fat 9%
Protein 27%
Carbohydrates 64%
Percent RDA:
Vitamin A 17%
Vitamin C 7%
Calcium 0%
Iron 8%

Nutrient	Amount per Serving	% Daily Value
Total Fat	2 g	4%
Saturated Fat	1 g	3%
Cholesterol	16 mg	5%
Sodium	605 mg	25%
Total Carbohydrate	39 g	13%
Dietary Fiber	1 g	4%
Sugars	0 g	
Protein	16 g	

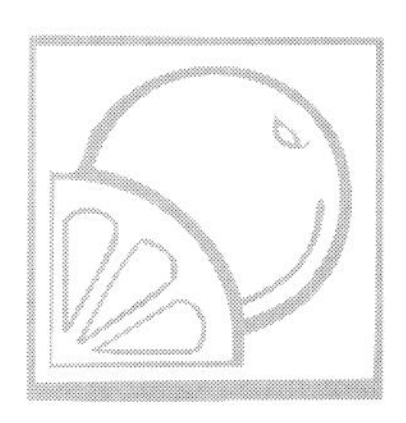

Spinach Salad

2 SERVINGS

1 cup fresh spinach, rinsed, dried, and roughly torn
½ cup canned mandarin orange sections
½ red onion, sliced thin

Dressing

⅛ cup balsamic vinegar
2 teaspoons honey
2 teaspoons mustard
4 bunches fresh basil, stems discarded and leaves roughly chopped

1. In a salad bowl, combine spinach, oranges, and onion.

2. Mix dressing ingredients thoroughly and toss with salad. Serve chilled.

PER SERVING
Calories 104
Calories from Fat 6
Percent Total Calories From:
Fat 5%
Protein 7%
Carbohydrates 88%
Percent RDA:
Vitamin A 49%
Vitamin C 53%
Calcium 0%
Iron 6%

Nutrient	Amount per Serving	% Daily Value
Total Fat	1 g	1%
Saturated Fat	0 g	0%
Cholesterol	0 mg	0%
Sodium	92 mg	4%
Total Carbohydrate	23 g	8%
Dietary Fiber	1 g	4%
Sugars	0 g	
Protein	2 g	

Jicama Salad

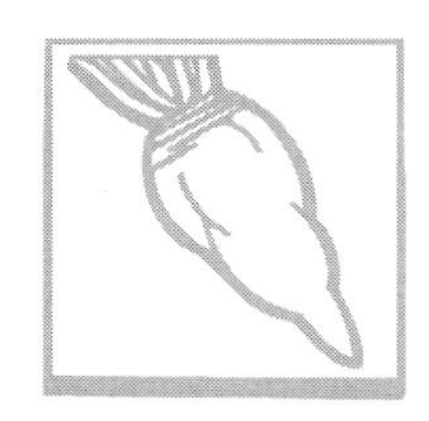

4 SERVINGS

½ jicama, peeled and cut into thin strips
2 carrots, peeled and cut into thin strips
1 pear, peeled and cut into thin strips
½ teaspoon minced fresh ginger
Juice of 2 limes
1 cup couscous, cooked
Pinch salt
Pinch pepper

1. In a large bowl, toss all ingredients. Serve cold.

PER SERVING
Calories 270
Calories from Fat 6
Percent Total Calories From:
Fat 2%
Protein 11%
Carbohydrates 86%
Percent RDA:
Vitamin A 23%
Vitamin C 54%
Calcium 0%
Iron 10%

Nutrient	Amount per Serving	% Daily Value
Total Fat	1 g	1%
Saturated Fat	0 g	0%
Cholesterol	0 mg	0%
Sodium	599 mg	25%
Total Carbohydrate	58 g	19%
Dietary Fiber	2 g	9%
Sugars	0 g	
Protein	8 g	

2 SERVINGS

Roast Vegetable Sandwich

Marinade

¼ cup olive oil
1 teaspoon fresh rosemary or lavender, chopped
1 teaspoon chopped garlic
1 teaspoon chopped fresh mint
2 tablespoons balsamic vinegar
1 teaspoon honey
Pinch salt
Pinch pepper

½ eggplant, sliced ⅛-inch thick
½ tomato, sliced ⅛-inch thick
½ red onion, sliced ⅛-inch thick
⅓ zucchini, sliced ⅛-inch thick
2 buns, whole wheat or multigrain
4 spinach leaves, rinsed and dried

PER SERVING
Calories 230
Calories from Fat 28
Percent Total Calories From:
Fat 12%
Protein 16%
Carbohydrates 72%
Percent RDA:
Vitamin A 158%
Vitamin C 82%
Calcium 0%
Iron 32%

Nutrient	Amount per Serving	% Daily Value
Total Fat	3 g	5%
Saturated Fat	1 g	3%
Cholesterol	2 mg	1%
Sodium	302 mg	13%
Total Carbohydrate	41 g	14%
Dietary Fiber	3 g	12%
Sugars	0 g	
Protein	9 g	

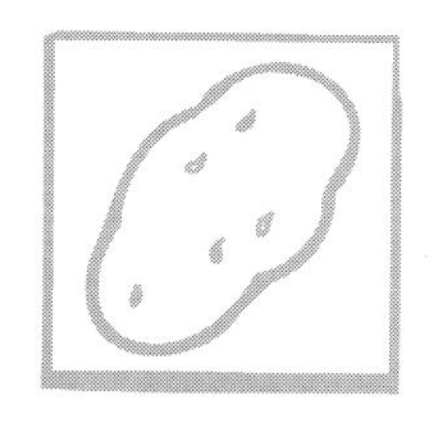

1. Preheat oven to 350 degrees F.

2. In a large bowl, combine all marinade ingredients and mix well.

3. Add eggplant, tomato, onion, and zucchini, toss, and let rest in marinade for 15 to 30 minutes.

4. Drain marinade and roast vegetables in oven for 10 to 15 minutes.

5. Stack vegetables in the bun with spinach, and continue to bake 5 more minutes.

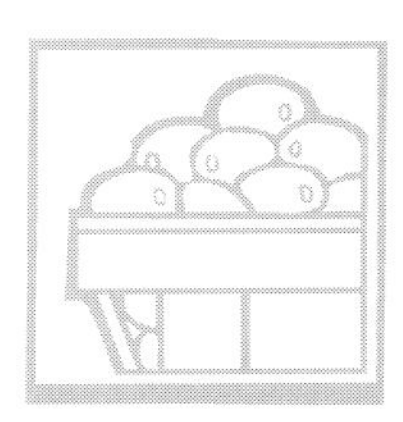

Seared Snapper Sandwich

2 SERVINGS

4 tablespoons olive oil
Pinch pepper
Pinch salt
3 sprigs fresh parsley, chopped
1 6-ounce snapper filet, cut in half
½ zucchini, cut into thin strips
¼ red onion, cut into thin strips
2 tablespoons capers, rinsed and drained
Juice of ½ lemon
1 tablespoon balsamic vinegar
2 whole grain buns

PER SERVING
Calories 395
Calories from Fat 176
Percent Total Calories From:
Fat 44%
Protein 27%
Carbohydrates 29%
Percent RDA:
Vitamin A 12%
Vitamin C 29%
Calcium 0%
Iron 20%

Nutrient	Amount per Serving	% Daily Value
Total Fat	20 g	30%
Saturated Fat	3 g	15%
Cholesterol	41 mg	14%
Sodium	379 mg	16%
Total Carbohydrate	29 g	10%
Dietary Fiber	1 g	4%
Sugars	0 g	
Protein	26 g	

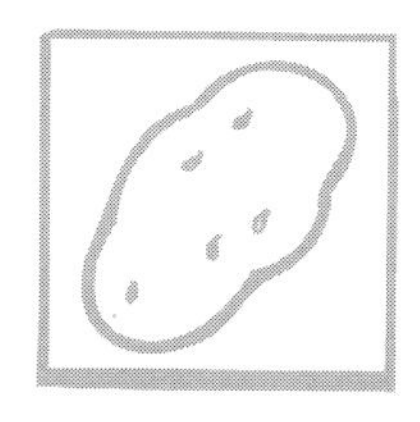

1. In a small bowl, combine 2 tablespoons olive oil, salt and pepper, and parsley. Brush mixture over both sides of fish filet.

2. Heat 1 tablespoon olive oil in a nonstick skillet. Add zucchini, onion, and capers, and cook for 3 minutes. Add lemon juice and vinegar and cook another 5 minutes. Set vegetables aside.

3. In the same skillet, heat the remaining tablespoon olive oil over medium heat. Sear filet approximately 3 minutes on each side.

4. Toast bun and place filet on bottom half, add vegetable mixture. Serve.

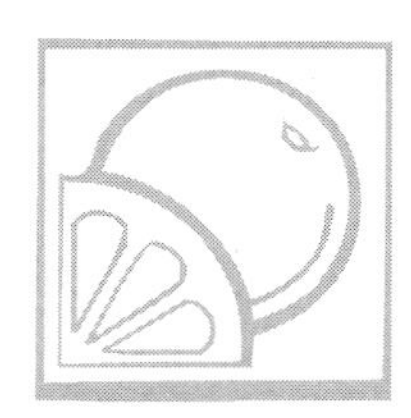

Blood Orange and Walnut Salad

4 SERVINGS

½ cup mixed greens
½ red onion, sliced thin
1 blood orange, peeled and segmented
¼ cup walnuts, halved

Dressing

⅓ cup canola oil
¼ cup champagne vinegar
2 tablespoons turbino
Pinch salt
Pinch pepper

1. In a salad bowl, combine mixed greens and onion.

2. In a small bowl, whisk all dressing ingredients together well.

3. Toss dressing with mixed greens and onion. Arrange salad on a plate and garnish with blood orange and walnuts. Serve chilled.

PER SERVING
Calories 274
Calories from Fat 207
Percent Total Calories From:
Fat 75%
Protein 3%
Carbohydrates 22%
Percent RDA:
Vitamin A 12%
Vitamin C 37%
Calcium 0%
Iron 3%

Nutrient	Amount per Serving	% Daily Value
Total Fat	23 g	35%
Saturated Fat	2 g	9%
Cholesterol	0 mg	0%
Sodium	585 mg	24%
Total Carbohydrate	15 g	5%
Dietary Fiber	1 g	3%
Sugars	0 g	
Protein	2 g	

Turkey Burger on Pita

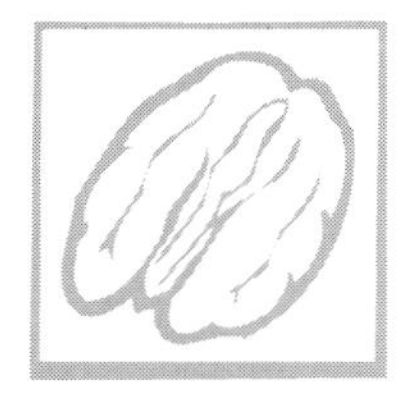

4 SERVINGS

1 pound ground turkey
1 cup dried chickpeas, cooked and smashed
½ cup cooked spinach, chopped
1 teaspoon ground coriander
1 teaspoon ground cumin
1 teaspoon dried sage
Pinch salt
Pinch pepper
1 ounce bean sprouts
4 pita breads, toasted

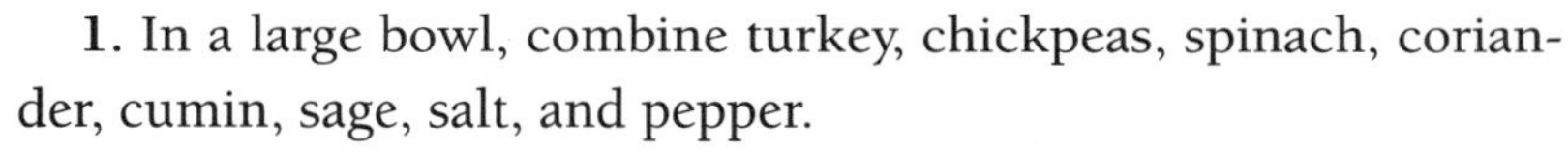

1. In a large bowl, combine turkey, chickpeas, spinach, coriander, cumin, sage, salt, and pepper.

2. Form into patties and grill until cooked through.

3. Serve with bean sprouts on a toasted pita.

PER SERVING
Calories 280
Calories from Fat 82
Percent Total Calories From:
Fat 29%
Protein 36%
Carbohydrates 35%
Percent RDA:
Vitamin A 11%
Vitamin C 9%
Calcium 0%
Iron 12%

Nutrient	Amount per Serving	% Daily Value
Total Fat	9 g	14%
Saturated Fat	2 g	12%
Cholesterol	83 mg	28%
Sodium	903 mg	38%
Total Carbohydrate	24 g	8%
Dietary Fiber	0 g	1%
Sugars	0 g	
Protein	25 g	

Indian Chicken Salad

4 SERVINGS

1 cup cooked and chopped chicken breasts
½ onion, sliced
½ cucumber, peeled, seeded, and chopped
1 tomato, seeded and chopped
½ cup plain nonfat yogurt
2 tablespoons curry powder
Pinch salt

1. In a medium bowl, mix all ingredients and chill. Serve cold

PER SERVING
Calories 106
Calories from Fat 34
Percent Total Calories From:
Fat 32%
Protein 40%
Carbohydrates 28%
Percent RDA:
Vitamin A 6%
Vitamin C 19%
Calcium 0%
Iron 8%

Nutrient	Amount per Serving	Value % Daily
Total Fat	4 g	6%
Saturated Fat	1 g	6%
Cholesterol	27 mg	9%
Sodium	621 mg	26%
Total Carbohydrate	7 g	2%
Dietary Fiber	1 g	4%
Sugars	0 g	
Protein	10 g	

Tuna Honduran

2 SERVINGS

1 bunch fresh cilantro, chopped
Juice of 2 limes
Pinch salt
Pinch pepper
1 6-ounce tuna steak
1 cup mixed salad greens
1 cup thinly sliced cabbage
Pinch salt
Pinch pepper
1 teaspoon ground cumin
Juice of 1 lemon

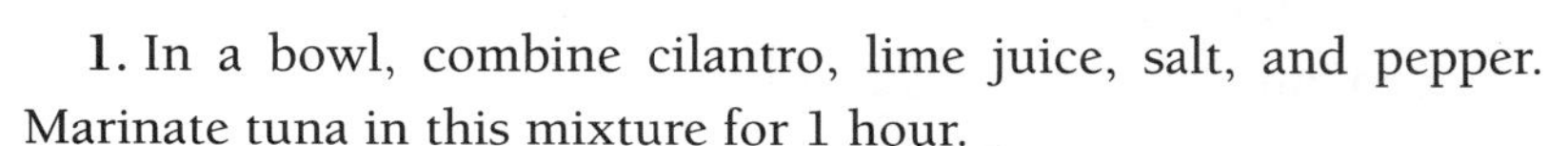

1. In a bowl, combine cilantro, lime juice, salt, and pepper. Marinate tuna in this mixture for 1 hour.

2. If baking tuna, preheat oven to 350 degrees F.

3. Grill tuna, or bake until medium rare, about 6 minutes.

4. Arrange mixed greens and cabbage on plate, season with salt, pepper, cumin, and lemon juice. Place tuna on bed of greens and serve.

PER SERVING
Calories 221
Calories from Fat 53
Percent Total Calories From:
Fat 24%
Protein 49%
Carbohydrates 27%
Percent RDA:
Vitamin A 84%
Vitamin C 105%
Calcium 0%
Iron 20%

Nutrient	Amount per Serving	Value % Daily
Total Fat	6 g	9%
Saturated Fat	1 g	7%
Cholesterol	40 mg	13%
Sodium	2385 mg	99%
Total Carbohydrate	15 g	5%
Dietary Fiber	1 g	5%
Sugars	0 g	
Protein	27 g	

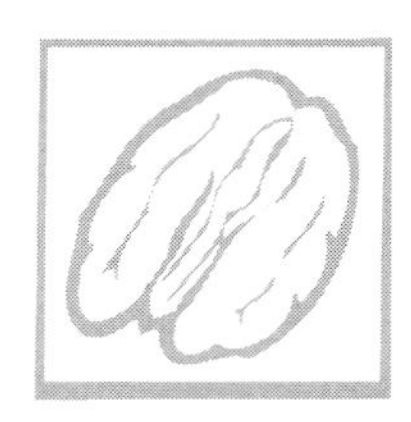

Three-Green, Citrus, Walnut, and Banana Salad

4 SERVINGS

Dressing

Juice and zest of 1 blood orange
Juice and zest of 1 lime
⅛ cup raw honey
Pinch ground cinnamon
½ teaspoon chopped fresh lavender (optional)

Salad

1 large ripe banana, peeled and sliced lengthwise
1 cup green leaf lettuce, washed, dried, and chilled
1 cup red leaf lettuce, washed, dried, and chilled
1 cup Bibb lettuce, washed, dried, and chilled
1 blood orange, peeled, segmented, or chopped
⅛ cup chopped walnuts

PER SERVING
Calories 144
Calories from Fat 25
Percent Total Calories From:
Fat 17%
Protein 6%
Carbohydrates 77%
Percent RDA:
Vitamin A 19%
Vitamin C 84%
Calcium 0%
Iron 7%

Nutrient	Amount per Serving	Value % Daily
Total Fat	3 g	4%
Saturated Fat	0 g	1%
Cholesterol	0 mg	0%
Sodium	6 mg	0%
Total Carbohydrate	28 g	9%
Dietary Fiber	1 g	5%
Sugars	0 g	
Protein	2 g	

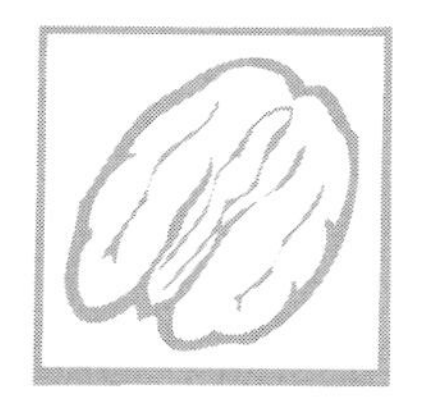

1. In a large bowl, combine dressing ingredients. Cover and refrigerate for 20 minutes.

2. Arrange the slices of banana on large chilled plate.

3. Toss remaining salad ingredients in dressing, shake excess dressing off, and arrange on top of bananas. Spoon some of remaining dressing around the salad.

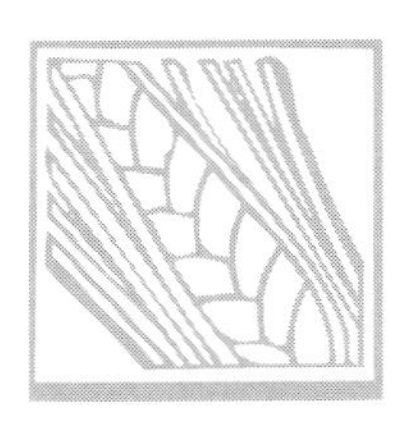

Spinach Crepes

6 SERVINGS

Crepes

⅔ cup soy milk
⅔ cup water
1 cup wheat flour
3 egg whites
Pinch salt
Oil

Filling

1 teaspoon olive oil
½ onion, diced
1 cup chopped spinach
Pinch nutmeg
2 cloves garlic, minced
1 cup nonfat cottage cheese

PER SERVING
Calories 148
Calories from Fat 30
Percent Total Calories From:
Fat 21%
Protein 26%
Carbohydrates 54%
Percent RDA:
Vitamin A 14%
Vitamin C 7%
Calcium 0%
Iron 4%

Nutrient	Amount per Serving	Value % Daily
Total Fat	3 g	5%
Saturated Fat	1 g	7%
Cholesterol	5 mg	2%
Sodium	568 mg	24%
Total Carbohydrate	20 g	7%
Dietary Fiber	0 g	1%
Sugars	0 g	
Protein	10 g	

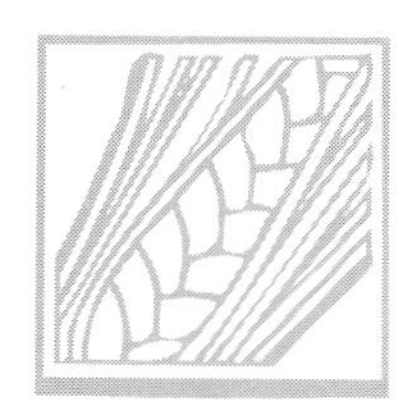

1. In a bowl, whisk soy milk and water into flour. Whisk in egg whites and salt.

2. Heat a 7-inch nonstick skillet, oil lightly.

3. Drop 2 tablespoons batter in skillet and roll pan to spread batter. Cook 30 seconds, flip crepe, and cook 30 seconds more.

4. Filling: In another pan, heat oil and cook onion until transparent. Add spinach, nutmeg, and garlic, cook for 5 minutes, and let cool.

5. Combine spinach mixture with cottage cheese and spoon into center of crepe. Fold crepe over filling and serve.

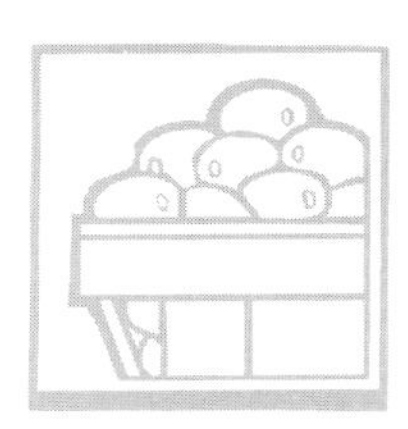

Portabella Mushroom and Spinach Sandwich

4 SERVINGS

3 tablespoons balsamic vinegar
1 tablespoon olive oil
Juice of ½ lemon
2 cloves garlic
1 teaspoon dried thyme
Pinch salt
Pinch pepper
8 ounces portabella mushroom, sliced
1 cup fresh spinach
½ cup sliced zucchini
½ cup sliced yellow squash
2 pita breads

PER SERVING
Calories 108
Calories from Fat 39
Percent Total Calories From:
Fat 36%
Protein 11%
Carbohydrates 53%
Percent RDA:
Vitamin A 21%
Vitamin C 18%
Calcium 0%
Iron 7%

Nutrient	Amount per Serving	Value % Daily
Total Fat	4 g	7%
Saturated Fat	1 g	3%
Cholesterol	0 mg	0%
Sodium	702 mg	29%
Total Carbohydrate	14 g	5%
Dietary Fiber	1 g	2%
Sugars	0 g	
Protein	3 g	

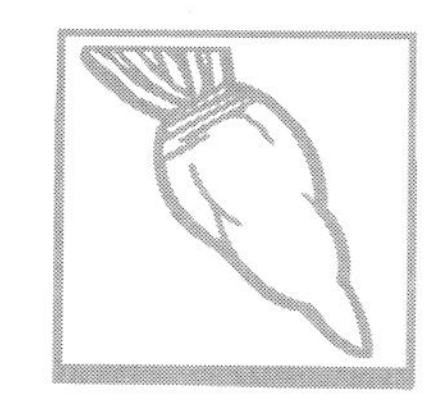

1. Preheat oven to 350 degrees F.

2. In a large bowl, mix vinegar, oil, lemon juice, garlic, thyme, salt, and pepper. Add sliced mushrooms, spinach, zucchini, and squash, toss to coat, and marinate for 30 minutes.

3. Drain vegetables, arrange in ovenproof casserole, and bake 8 to 10 minutes, until tender. As an alternative, you may grill the vegetables until tender.

4. Toast pita, slice in half, stuff with vegetables, and serve.

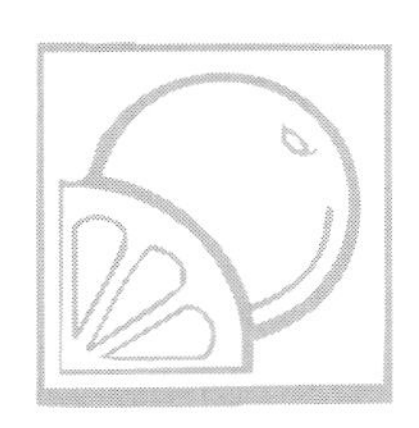

Chicken Orange Salad

4 SERVINGS

Dressing

¼ cup olive oil
½ cup white vinegar
Juice of 3 oranges
½ cup Curry Powder (see recipe, page 50)
2 oranges, sectioned
Pinch salt
Pinch pepper
Pinch turbino

Salad

1 head romaine lettuce, torn
1 cup fresh spinach
1 cup cooked and diced chicken

1. In a bowl, whisk oil and vinegar. Add remaining dressing ingredients, being careful not to break orange sections. Refrigerate 45 minutes.

2. Wash lettuce and spinach and drain well. Combine with chicken and toss with dressing. Serve chilled.

PER SERVING
Calories 290
Calories from Fat 158
Percent Total Calories From:
Fat 54%
Protein 5%
Carbohydrates 40%
Percent RDA:
Vitamin A 35%
Vitamin C 160%
Calcium 0%
Iron 26%

Nutrient	Amount per Serving	Value % Daily
Total Fat	18 g	27%
Saturated Fat	2 g	11%
Cholesterol	0 mg	0%
Sodium	601 mg	25%
Total Carbohydrate	29 g	10%
Dietary Fiber	3 g	12%
Sugars	0 g	
Protein	4 g	

Calamari Salad

4 SERVINGS

2 tablespoons olive oil
6 ounces calamari, sliced into ⅛-inch tubes and tentacles
2 cups fresh spinach, stems and veins removed
Balsamic vinegar to taste
Dash olive oil

Dressing

2 plum tomatoes, diced
½ cup leeks, sliced into thin rings
½ cup onions, diced
½ tablespoon capers
Juice of 1 lemon
1 tablespoon basil

1. In a large bowl, combine dressing ingredients.

2. In a nonstick sauté pan, heat oil over medium heat. Sauté calamari quickly, approximately 2 minutes.

3. Combine calamari with dressing and mix well.

4. Arrange spinach on plate. Drizzle light amount of balsamic vinegar and olive oil on spinach. Place calamari and dressing on spinach and serve.

PER SERVING
Calories 102
Calories from Fat 72
Percent Total Calories From:
Fat 71%
Protein 6%
Carbohydrates 24%
Percent RDA:
Vitamin A 38%
Vitamin C 31%
Calcium 0%
Iron 7%

Nutrient	Amount per Serving	Value % Daily
Total Fat	8 g	12%
Saturated Fat	1 g	5%
Cholesterol	0 mg	0%
Sodium	41 mg	2%
Total Carbohydrate	6 g	2%
Dietary Fiber	1 g	3%
Sugars	0 g	
Protein	1 g	

Grilled Chicken Breast with Banana and Grape Sauce

2 SERVINGS

1 teaspoon vanilla extract
1 teaspoon ground cinnamon
Pinch nutmeg
1 tablespoon honey
½ teaspoon cayenne pepper
2 drops olive oil
2 whole chicken breasts, skinless
1 banana, cut lengthwise
Sprig fresh rosemary, for garnish

Sauce

1 cup white grape juice
1 teaspoon cornstarch, mixed with a little grape juice
2 tablespoons white wine
½ cup seedless grapes

PER SERVING
Calories 566
Calories from Fat 142
Percent Total Calories From:
Fat 25%
Protein 41%
Carbohydrates 33%
Percent RDA:
Vitamin A 9%
Vitamin C 62%
Calcium 0%
Iron 18%

Nutrient	Amount per Serving	Value % Daily
Total Fat	16 g	24%
Saturated Fat	5 g	24%
Cholesterol	159 mg	53%
Sodium	138 mg	6%
Total Carbohydrate	46 g	15%
Dietary Fiber	1 g	4%
Sugars	0 g	
Protein	57 g	

1. In a bowl, combine vanilla, cinnamon, nutmeg, honey, cayenne pepper, and olive oil. Mix well, coat chicken with mixture, and refrigerate for 1 hour. Preheat grill.

2. Make the sauce: In a small saucepan, bring grape juice to a boil. Add cornstarch mixture and reduce heat to simmer. When sauce thickens, add wine and grapes. Simmer 2 minutes.

3. Grill chicken until done. Grill banana 1 minute on each side.

4. Put chicken on plate and spoon sauce over it to one side. Place grilled banana on the other side of chicken. Garnish with sprigs of fresh rosemary.

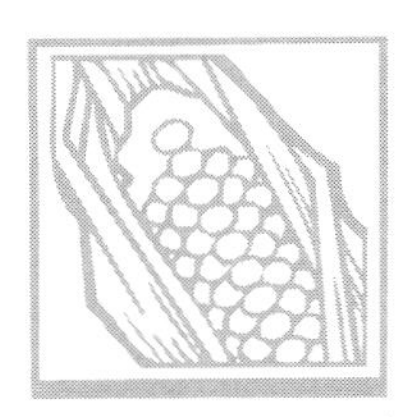

Sea Bass Tostada

2 SERVINGS

2 4-ounce sea bass steaks
Pinch salt
Pinch pepper
Pinch cumin
Juice of 1 lime
1 teaspoon olive oil
½ white onion, chopped
2 green onions, sliced thin
½ cup frozen corn kernels
1 tablespoon chopped fresh cilantro
Pinch salt
Pinch pepper
4 whole wheat tortillas

1. Preheat oven to 350 degrees F.

2. Sprinkle fish with salt, pepper, and cumin and place filets on baking sheet. Sprinkle fish with some of the lime juice and bake for about 8 minutes, or until done.

PER SERVING
Calories 110
Calories from Fat 24
Percent Total Calories From:
Fat 22%
Protein 41%
Carbohydrates 37%
Percent RDA:
Vitamin A 3%
Vitamin C 15%
Calcium 0%
Iron 4%

Nutrient	Amount per Serving	Value % Daily
Total Fat	3 g	4%
Saturated Fat	0 g	2%
Cholesterol	23 mg	8%
Sodium	1203 mg	50%
Total Carbohydrate	10 g	3%
Dietary Fiber	1 g	2%
Sugars	0 g	
Protein	11 g	

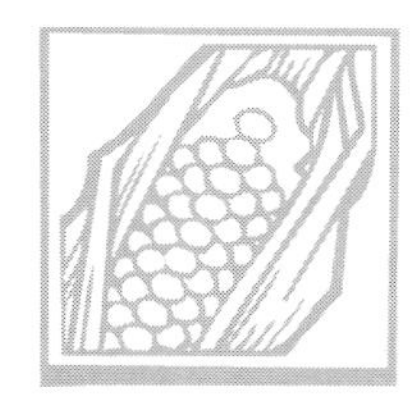

3. Heat olive oil in a sauté pan, add onions and corn, and stir constantly until tender.

4. Add cilantro, remaining lime juice, salt, and pepper, stir, and pour into a large mixing bowl.

5. Heat tortillas in the oven until warm, about 2 or 3 minutes.

6. Flake cooked filet into onion and corn mixture and mix lightly.

7. Place 1 tortilla on plate, top with some filling, cover with second tortilla, top with remaining filling, repeat with remaining tortillas and filling, and serve.

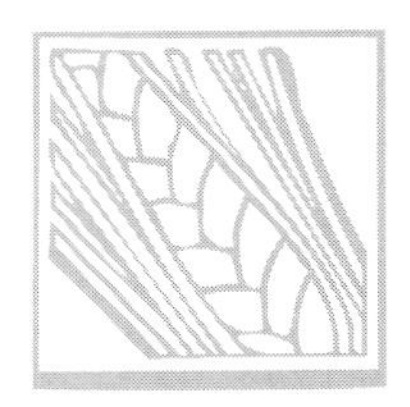

Spinach Eggplant Pizza

4 SERVINGS

1 cup fresh spinach
2 cloves garlic
2 tablespoons olive oil
Pinch salt
Pinch pepper
4 whole wheat pita breads
1 small eggplant, peeled and diced
1 tablespoon Parmesan cheese

1. Preheat oven to 350 degrees F.

2. In a blender, puree spinach and garlic. Add olive oil to form a paste and season with salt and pepper.

3. Spread paste on pita and place diced eggplant on top. Sprinkle with Parmesan cheese.

4. Bake until golden brown, about 10 minutes.

PER SERVING
Calories 219
Calories from Fat 81
Percent Total Calories From:
Fat 37%
Protein 11%
Carbohydrates 52%
Percent RDA:
Vitamin A 20%
Vitamin C 10%
Calcium 0%
Iron 6%

Nutrient	Amount per Serving	Value % Daily
Total Fat	9 g	14%
Saturated Fat	1 g	7%
Cholesterol	1 mg	0%
Sodium	841 mg	35%
Total Carbohydrate	28 g	9%
Dietary Fiber	1 g	5%
Sugars	0 g	
Protein	6 g	

Pasta and Asparagus

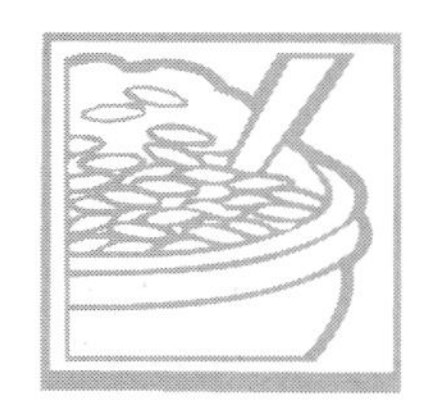

4 SERVINGS

1 tablespoon olive oil
1 cup chopped white onions
3 cloves garlic, sliced thin
1 cup chopped spinach
5 asparagus, sliced on the bias
Pinch red pepper flakes
½ cup white wine
Juice of 1 lemon
Pinch salt
1 cup pasta, cooked and well drained

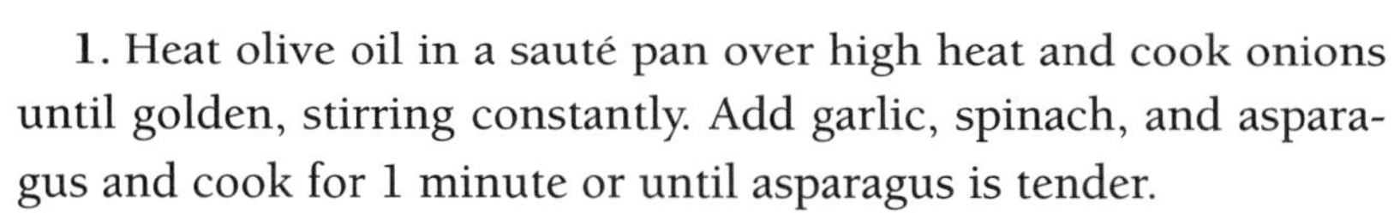

1. Heat olive oil in a sauté pan over high heat and cook onions until golden, stirring constantly. Add garlic, spinach, and asparagus and cook for 1 minute or until asparagus is tender.

2. Sprinkle in red pepper flakes and add wine. Simmer until reduced by half. Add lemon juice and salt to taste.

3. Put pasta in a serving bowl, toss with sauce, and serve.

PER SERVING
Calories 136
Calories from Fat 40
Percent Total Calories From:
- Fat 29%
- Protein 10%
- Carbohydrates 46%

Percent RDA:
- Vitamin A 22%
- Vitamin C 34%
- Calcium 0%
- Iron 8%

Nutrient	Amount per Serving	Value % Daily
Total Fat	4 g	7%
Saturated Fat	1 g	3%
Cholesterol	12 mg	4%
Sodium	601 mg	25%
Total Carbohydrate	16 g	5%
Dietary Fiber	1 g	3%
Sugars	0 g	
Protein	4 g	

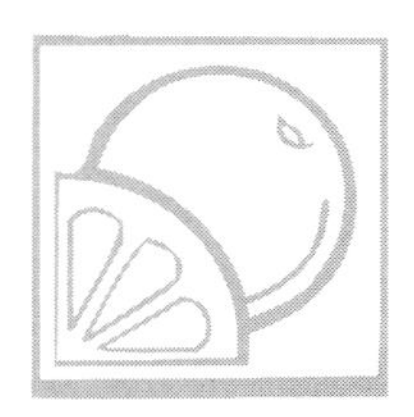

4 SERVINGS

Citrus Salad

2 oranges, peeled and segmented
1 grapefruit, peeled and segmented
3 tablespoons honey
1 bunch fresh mint, chopped
1 cup chopped romaine lettuce

1. In a bowl, toss citrus segments in a bowl with honey and mint.

2. Arrange on lettuce and serve.

PER SERVING
Calories 110
Calories from Fat 2
Percent Total Calories From:
Fat 2%
Protein 4%
Carbohydrates 94%
Percent RDA:
Vitamin A 7%
Vitamin C 99%
Calcium 0%
Iron 2%

Nutrient	Amount per Serving	Value % Daily
Total Fat	0 g	0%
Saturated Fat	0 g	0%
Cholesterol	0 mg	0%
Sodium	2 mg	0%
Total Carbohydrate	26 g	9%
Dietary Fiber	0 g	2%
Sugars	0 g	
Protein	1 g	

Spinach Salmon

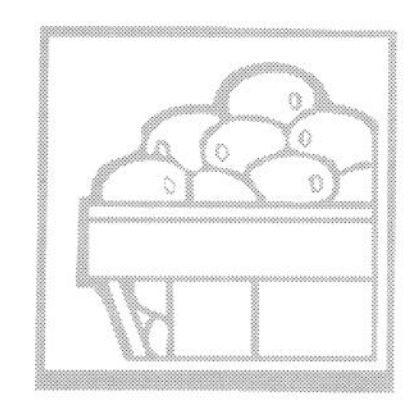

2 SERVINGS

2 whole wheat pita breads
Olive oil
1 6-ounce salmon filet, sliced thin
½ cup fresh spinach
½ onion, chopped
2 tablespoons chopped garlic
4 tablespoons fresh thyme
Pinch salt
Pinch pepper

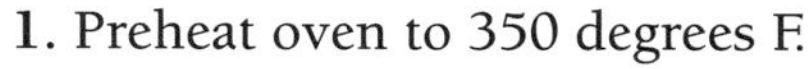

1. Preheat oven to 350 degrees F.

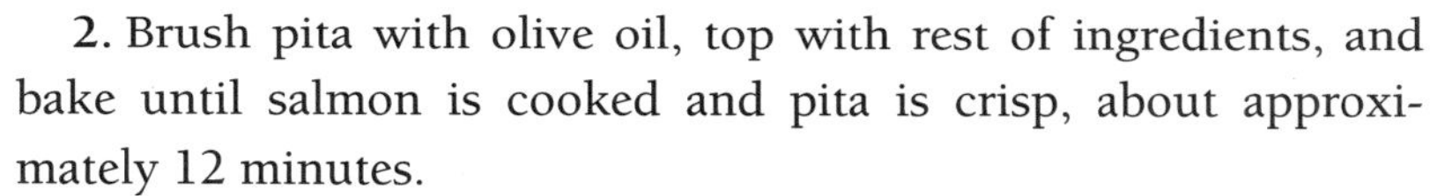

2. Brush pita with olive oil, top with rest of ingredients, and bake until salmon is cooked and pita is crisp, about approximately 12 minutes.

PER SERVING
Calories 300
Calories from Fat 71
Percent Total Calories From:
Fat 24%
Protein 26%
Carbohydrates 50%
Percent RDA:
Vitamin A 26%
Vitamin C 21%
Calcium 0%
Iron 68%

Nutrient	Amount per Serving	Value % Daily
Total Fat	8 g	12%
Saturated Fat	2 g	8%
Cholesterol	35 mg	12%
Sodium	590 mg	25%
Total Carbohydrate	37 g	12%
Dietary Fiber	3 g	10%
Sugars	0 g	
Protein	20 g	

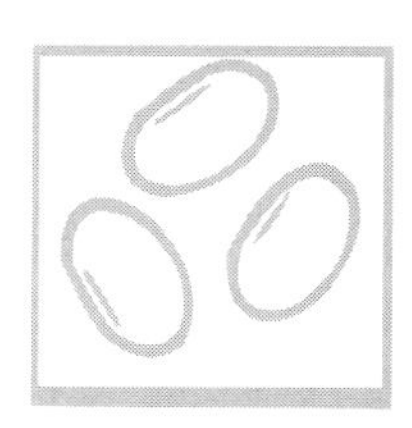

Chicken Pizza

4 SERVINGS

1 tablespoon ground cumin
5 tablespoons olive oil
Juice of 1 lemon
1 bunch fresh cilantro, chopped
1 whole chicken breast
¼ cup cooked black beans
2 whole wheat pita breads
Kernels from 1 ear of fresh corn, or ⅓ cup frozen
2 green onions, sliced thin
½ red onion, diced
Pinch salt
Pinch pepper

1. In a bowl, combine cumin, 1 tablespoon olive oil, lemon, and cilantro. Marinate chicken breast in mixture for 1 hour. Grill or sauté chicken until fully cooked. Let cool, then chop into large chunks.

2. Preheat oven to 350 degrees F.

PER SERVING
Calories 358
Calories from Fat 215
Percent Total Calories From:
Fat 60%
Protein 20%
Carbohydrates 20%
Percent RDA:
Vitamin A 2%
Vitamin C 17%
Calcium 0%
Iron 12%

Nutrient	Amount per Serving	Value % Daily
Total Fat	24 g	37%
Saturated Fat	4 g	18%
Cholesterol	40 mg	13%
Sodium	752 mg	31%
Total Carbohydrate	18 g	6%
Dietary Fiber	1 g	3%
Sugars	0 g	
Protein	18 g	

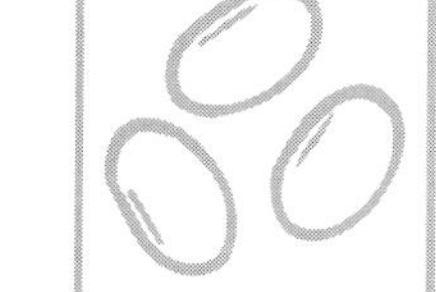

3. In a blender, puree black beans and remaining 4 tablespoons olive oil.

4. Put pitas on a baking sheet, spread with black beans, and top with chicken, corn, onions, and salt and pepper.

5. Bake until pita is crisp, about 10 minutes. Serve warm.

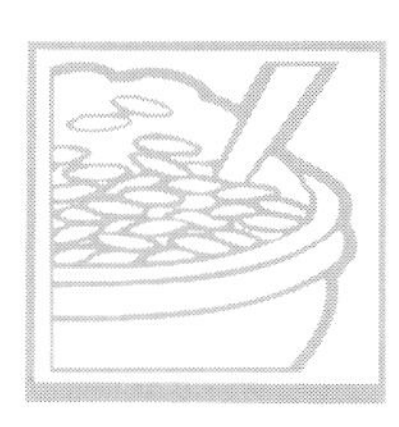

Beef and Pasta Soup

8 SERVINGS

1 pound beef bones, trimmed of fat
1 tablespoon olive oil
1 onion, chopped
1 carrot, chopped
2 stalks celery, chopped
1 bay leaf
3 sprigs fresh thyme
5 black peppercorns
4 allspice berries
2 cloves garlic
1 cup pasta, partially cooked
1 lemon, sliced

1. Preheat oven to 350 degrees F.

2. Place beef bones in roasting pan. Roast in oven until browned, about 25 minutes.

3. Heat oil in a large stockpot and cook vegetables for 5 minutes on medium heat.

PER SERVING
Calories 65
Calories from Fat 21
Percent Total Calories From:
Fat 32%
Protein 10%
Carbohydrates 59%
Percent RDA:
Vitamin A 51%
Vitamin C 11%
Calcium 0%
Iron 7%

Nutrient	Amount per Serving	Value % Daily
Total Fat	2 g	4%
Saturated Fat	0 g	2%
Cholesterol	6 mg	2%
Sodium	7 mg	0%
Total Carbohydrate	10 g	3%
Dietary Fiber	1 g	3%
Sugars	0 g	
Protein	2 g	

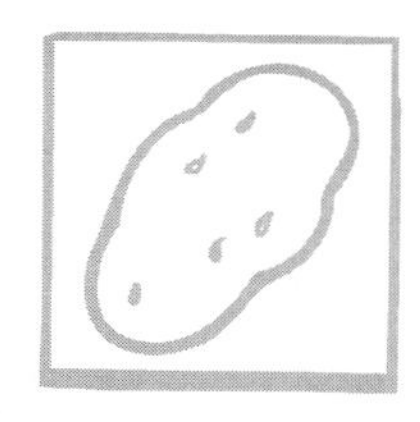

4. Add beef bones and remaining ingredients except pasta and lemon, and cover with 8 cups of cold water.

5. Simmer 4 to 8 hours, skimming foam off top of broth. When done, strain broth into container, cool, and refrigerate for use later.

6. When ready to serve, add any organic pasta to beef broth, heat, and cook until pasta is done. Add 2 lemon slices and serve.

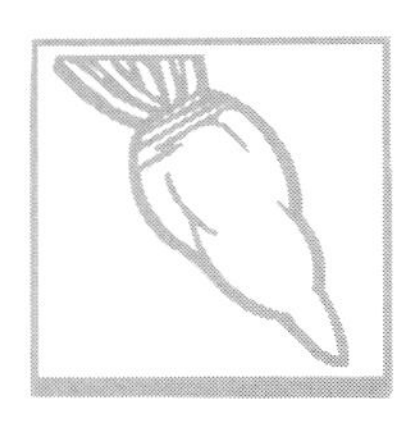

Tahini Turkey Pizza

4 SERVINGS

1 pound ground turkey
1 teaspoon dried sage
1 teaspoon minced garlic
Pinch salt
Pinch pepper
1 leek, sliced thin
4 tablespoons tahini paste
4 whole wheat pita breads
2 tablespoons grated Parmesan cheese

1. Preheat oven to 350 degrees F.
2. In a large bowl, combine turkey, sage, garlic, salt, and pepper.
3. In a nonstick sauté pan, brown turkey mixture with leeks and tahini.
4. Top pita with turkey mixture, sprinkle cheese on top, and bake for 5 to 10 minutes.

PER SERVING
Calories 300
Calories from Fat 90
Percent Total Calories From:
- Fat 30%
- Protein 35%
- Carbohydrates 35%

Percent RDA:
- Vitamin A 1%
- Vitamin C 7%
- Calcium 0%
- Iron 12%

Nutrient	Amount per Serving	Value % Daily
Total Fat	10 g	15%
Saturated Fat	3 g	15%
Cholesterol	85 mg	28%
Sodium	960 mg	40%
Total Carbohydrate	26 g	9%
Dietary Fiber	1 g	3%
Sugars	0 g	
Protein	26 g	

Pumpkin Seed Salad

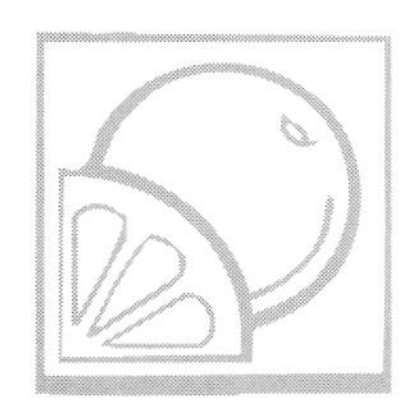

4 SERVINGS

Dressing

2 kiwis, peeled
4 tablespoons champagne vinegar
2 tablespoons honey
1 bunch fresh mint, chopped

Salad

2 cups chopped red leaf lettuce
1 orange, peeled and segmented
⅛ cup pumpkin seeds, shelled
⅛ cup flax seeds

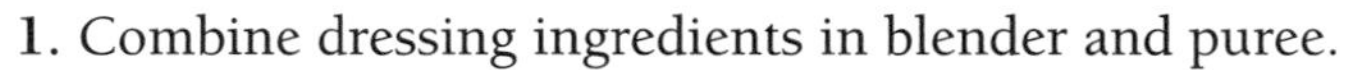

1. Combine dressing ingredients in blender and puree.

2. In a salad bowl, toss lettuce with dressing. Arrange on a plate and garnish with orange segments, pumpkin seeds, and flax seeds. Serve chilled.

PER SERVING
Calories 89
Calories from Fat 6
Percent Total Calories From:
- Fat 6%
- Protein 5%
- Carbohydrates 88%

Percent RDA:
- Vitamin A 5%
- Vitamin C 94%
- Calcium 0%
- Iron 3%

Nutrient	Amount per Serving	Value % Daily
Total Fat	1 g	1%
Saturated Fat	0 g	0%
Cholesterol	0 mg	0%
Sodium	4 mg	0%
Total Carbohydrate	20 g	7%
Dietary Fiber	1 g	5%
Sugars	0 g	
Protein	1 g	

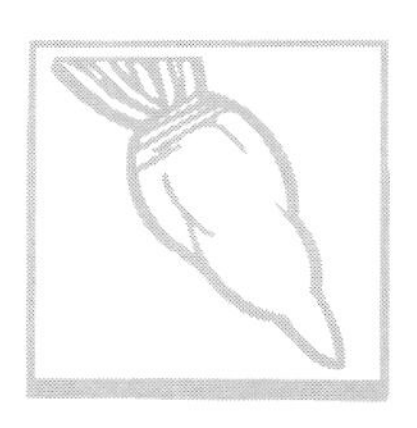

Chicken Gumbo L'Herb

10 SERVINGS

1 medium cabbage
1 pound mustard greens, chopped
1 pound collard greens, chopped
1 pound turnip greens, chopped
1 pound fresh spinach, chopped
4 carrots, sliced
1 pound turnips, peeled and diced
1 bunch fresh parsley
½ onion, chopped
1 bunch green onions, chopped
2 cloves garlic, diced
4 stalks celery, chopped
Pinch salt
Pinch pepper
1 teaspoon dried thyme
3 teaspoons gumbo file
3 bay leaves
½ quart chicken stock
1 pound chicken, diced

PER SERVING
Calories 179
Calories from Fat 14
Percent Total Calories From:
Fat 8%
Protein 19%
Carbohydrates 73%
Percent RDA:
Vitamin A 384%
Vitamin C 258%
Calcium 0%
Iron 29%

Nutrient	Amount per Serving	Value % Daily
Total Fat	2 g	2%
Saturated Fat	0 g	2%
Cholesterol	0 mg	0%
Sodium	710 mg	30%
Total Carbohydrate	33 g	11%
Dietary Fiber	6 g	23%
Sugars	0 g	
Protein	9 g	

1. Wash all greens and drain well. Place in large pot with carrots and turnips; add enough water to cover greens.

2. Bring to a boil, reduce heat, and simmer for 20 minutes.

3. Add remaining ingredients and simmer an additional 45 minutes. Serve gumbo as is or over rice.

Spinach Lasagna

8 SERVINGS

8 ounces dried lasagna noodles

Filling

1 cup nonfat cottage cheese
8 ounces fresh spinach, washed and chopped
15 ounces canned canellini beans, drained and rinsed
2 tablespoons chopped fresh oregano
2 tablespoons chopped fresh basil

Sauce

1 8-ounce can chicken broth
1 bouquet garni (3 black peppercorns, 3 stems fresh parsley, 2 sprigs fresh thyme, 1 clove tied in a clean muslin bag)
1½ tablespoons cornstarch, mixed with 3 tablespoons water
½ nonfat plain yogurt

1. Cook lasagna noodles according to package directions. Drain, rinse, and keep noodles in cool water until ready to use.

2. Make the filling: In a large bowl, combine cottage cheese, spinach, beans, oregano, and basil.

PER SERVING
Calories 342
Calories from Fat 26
Percent Total Calories From:
Fat 8%
Protein 25%
Carbohydrates 67%
Percent RDA:
Vitamin A 41%
Vitamin C 18%
Calcium 0%
Iron 41%

Nutrient	Amount per Serving	Value % Daily
Total Fat	3 g	4%
Saturated Fat	1 g	6%
Cholesterol	6 mg	2%
Sodium	316 mg	13%
Total Carbohydrate	57 g	19%
Dietary Fiber	4 g	15%
Sugars	0 g	
Protein	22 g	

3. Make the sauce: In a saucepan, heat chicken broth and bouquet garni. Bring to a boil and add cornstarch mixture. Reduce heat and simmer, stirring constantly until thickened. Remove bouquet garni and let cool until warm. Add yogurt and set aside.

4. Preheat oven to 350 degrees F.

5. Lay lasagna noodles flat on a cutting board. Form ⅓ cup filling into a ball. Place ball on end of noodle and roll. Repeat with all noodles.

6. Pour half of the sauce in the bottom of an ungreased 9 × 13-inch baking pan. Place lasagna rolls in pan, seam side down. Cover with remaining sauce. Cover pan with aluminum foil and bake for 30 minutes.

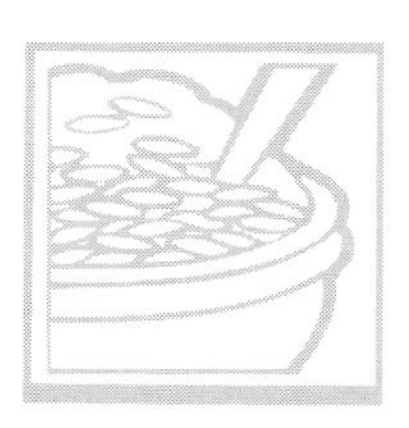

Red Beans and Rice with Pork Tenderloin

6 SERVINGS

2 cups dried red beans, rinsed and drained
½ small onion, diced
2 stalks celery, chopped
1 bay leaf
1 teaspoon dried thyme
4 cups chicken stock
Dash vinegar
Dash hot sauce
Pinch salt
Pinch pepper
1 teaspoon olive oil
Dash salt
Dash cracked black pepper
6 slices 1½-inch-thick (6 ounces) pork tenderloin
1 cup white rice, cooked

PER SERVING
Calories 376
Calories from Fat 25
Percent Total Calories From:
Fat 7%
Protein 20%
Carbohydrates 73%
Percent RDA:
Vitamin A 2%
Vitamin C 7%
Calcium 0%
Iron 30%

Nutrient	Amount per Serving	Value % Daily
Total Fat	3 g	4%
Saturated Fat	1 g	3%
Cholesterol	9 mg	3%
Sodium	1452 mg	61%
Total Carbohydrate	69 g	23%
Dietary Fiber	4 g	16%
Sugars	0 g	
Protein	19 g	

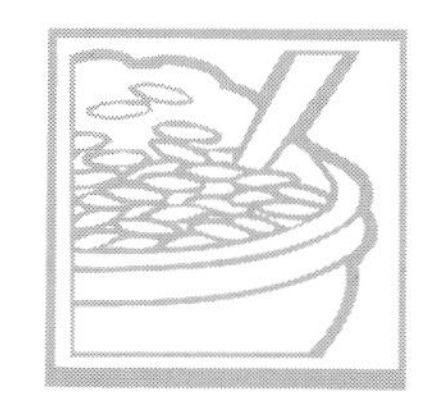

1. In a large pot, combine beans, onion, celery, bay leaf, thyme, and chicken stock. Simmer until beans are cooked.

2. Cook rice according to directions.

3. Remove half the beans and liquid, let cool, and puree in blender. Add back to pot, mix well, and season with vinegar, hot sauce, salt, and pepper.

4. In a small bowl, mix oil, salt, and pepper. Brush on pork. Cook pork in a shallow pan over medium heat until done, approximately 4 minutes on each side.

5. Put rice on plate, serve beans over rice, and add 1 slice of pork per serving.

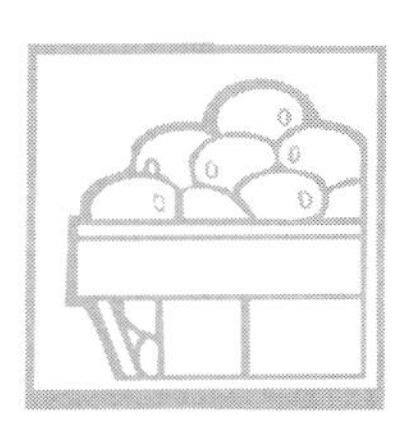

Home-cured Salmon

20 SERVINGS

2 2-pound salmon filets
½ cup vodka, pepper flavor
2 tablespoons caraway seeds
½ cup chopped fresh dill
1 teaspoon fresh ground black pepper
⅓ cup turbino
⅓ cup kosher salt

1. Put salmon in a nonaluminum pan and moisten with pepper vodka. Sprinkle caraway, dill, and pepper on both sides of filets. Combine turbino and salt and liberally coat fish.

2. Cover fish with plastic wrap and lightly weight with another pan. Refrigerate for 4 days, turning fish once a day and replacing the weight.

3. On the fifth day, the salmon should be cured. Slice and serve with bitter greens and sweet and spicy mustard sauce.

PER SERVING
Calories 108
Calories from Fat 38
Percent Total Calories From:
Fat 35%
Protein 51%
Carbohydrates 3%
Percent RDA:
Vitamin A 1%
Vitamin C 0%
Calcium 0%
Iron 7%

Nutrient	Amount per Serving	Value % Daily
Total Fat	4 g	6%
Saturated Fat	1 g	5%
Cholesterol	37 mg	12%
Sodium	2241 mg	93%
Total Carbohydrate	1 g	0%
Dietary Fiber	0 g	1%
Sugars	0 g	
Protein	14 g	

Root Vegetable Salad

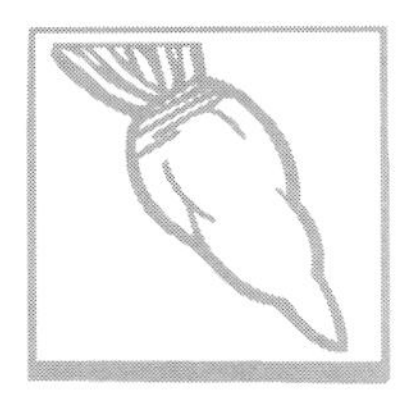

4 SERVINGS

- 2 cups mixed torn salad greens, endive, spinach, watercress, and lettuce
- 2 carrots, peeled and sliced lengthwise
- 1 beet, sliced
- 1 turnip, sliced
- 6 ounces dried garbanzo beans, cooked
- 1 green onion, sliced
- 3 radishes, sliced
- 2 tablespoons honey
- Juice of 1 lime

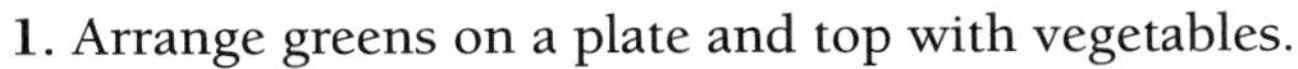

1. Arrange greens on a plate and top with vegetables.

2. In a small bowl, combine honey and lime. Pour dressing over salad and serve.

PER SERVING
Calories 165
Calories from Fat 13
Percent Total Calories From:
- Fat 8%
- Protein 14%
- Carbohydrates 78%

Percent RDA:
- Vitamin A 244%
- Vitamin C 53%
- Calcium 0%
- Iron 13%

Nutrient	Amount per Serving	Value % Daily
Total Fat	1 g	2%
Saturated Fat	0 g	1%
Cholesterol	0 mg	0%
Sodium	169 mg	7%
Total Carbohydrate	32 g	11%
Dietary Fiber	2 g	9%
Sugars	0 g	
Protein	6 g	

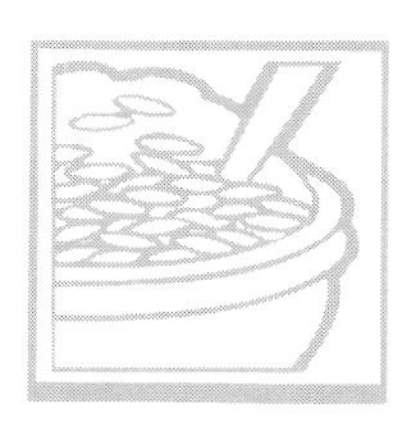

Chicken Soup with Wild Rice

8 SERVINGS

6 cups chicken stock
1 whole chicken breast, boned, skinned, and diced
½ head cabbage, cored and sliced
1 carrot, peeled and sliced
1 onion, peeled and sliced
1 turnip, peeled and diced
1 parsnip, peeled and diced
1 tablespoon dried tarragon
1 tablespoon dried thyme
⅓ cup wild rice, cooked
Pinch salt
Pinch pepper
2 green onions, sliced

1. Bring chicken stock to a boil in a large pot. Add diced chicken and boil for 1 minute. Reduce heat to simmer.

2. Add all vegetables except green onion, and simmer for 1 hour. Add more chicken stock if needed.

3. Add tarragon, thyme, and rice. Simmer for 10 minutes. Salt and pepper to taste. Garnish with green onion and serve.

PER SERVING
Calories 134
Calories from Fat 27
Percent Total Calories From:
Fat 20%
Protein 32%
Carbohydrates 48%
Percent RDA:
Vitamin A 54%
Vitamin C 58%
Calcium 0%
Iron 11%

Nutrient	Amount per Serving	Value % Daily
Total Fat	3 g	5%
Saturated Fat	1 g	4%
Cholesterol	20 mg	7%
Sodium	1431 mg	60%
Total Carbohydrate	16 g	5%
Dietary Fiber	1 g	5%
Sugars	0 g	
Protein	11 g	

Chapter 5

DINNER

Healthful Dining, Pain-Free Nights

IF YOUR HOUSEHOLD IS ANYTHING LIKE OURS, DINNER-time is nothing short of traumatic. What to make, how quickly can I get the food on the table, how much time do I have to spend cleaning up, and will everyone enjoy it after all that work?

But are these really the questions you should be asking yourself? We think it's more important to ask, "What can I do to make myself feel better; what can I do to help myself have a restful and pain-free night, and what can I do to make sure that tomorrow is off to a better start?"

"What can I do to make myself feel better; what can I do to help myself have a restful and pain-free night, and what can I do to make sure that tomorrow is off to a better start?"

As we've discussed earlier, some foods that are good for you and some foods are not. In this chapter we offer you thirty healthful, delicious, and appetizing dinners created by Chef Neal. These great recipes are not only good for you, but they are also tasty, interesting to prepare, and relatively simple to clean up.

We know that dinnertime is often a hectic time of the day, and sometimes you don't always have the time, strength, energy, or desire to make that four- or five-course evening meal. In the perfect world, lunch would be the major meal, with a very light meal at dinnertime. Consequently, if you so choose to once in awhile, you can eat our dinner recipes for lunch instead. But do try to follow our diet as to timing as well and eat what we recommend for lunch at lunch time.

We worked to create an anti-arthritis diet that works with your active lifestyle, one you can live with and enjoy. We hope these recipes will help you with a wholesome and nutritious start for the evening, and keep you in the healthful cycle of improved health, improved nutrition, and, hopefully, decreased arthritis pain relief. Bon appetit!

Winter Vegetable Roast

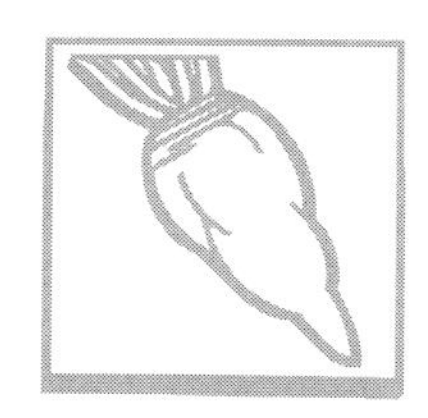

6 SERVINGS

1½ tablespoons olive oil
1 rutabaga, peeled and diced
2 carrots, peeled and diced
12 pearl onions
1 zucchini, sliced
2 beets with greens attached, peeled and diced
½ cup chicken stock
¼ teaspoon dried thyme
¼ teaspoon dried rosemary
¼ teaspoon dried tarragon
Pinch salt
Pinch pepper

1. Preheat oven to 400 degrees F.

2. In a large baking dish, combine all ingredients. Bake about 40 minutes or until vegetables are tender. Serve over rice.

PER SERVING
Calories 124
Calories from Fat 39
Percent Total Calories From:
Fat 32%
Protein 9%
Carbohydrates 59%
Percent RDA:
Vitamin A 137%
Vitamin C 64%
Calcium 0%
Iron 8%

Nutrient	Amount per Serving	% Daily Value
Total Fat	4 g	7%
Saturated Fat	1 g	3%
Cholesterol	0 mg	0%
Sodium	572 mg	24%
Total Carbohydrate	18 g	6%
Dietary Fiber	2 g	8%
Sugars	0 g	
Protein	3 g	

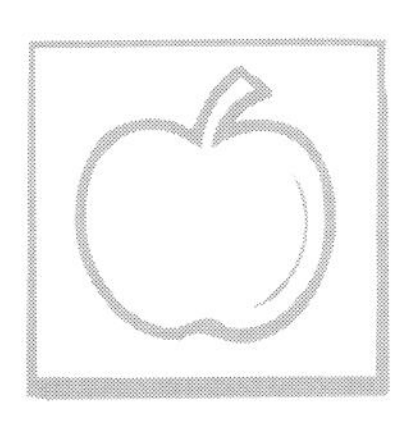

Baked Turkey Cutlets

4 SERVINGS

3 tablespoons Dijon mustard
2½ tablespoons lemon juice
1½ tablespoons turbino
1 tablespoon dried tarragon
1 teaspoon ground sage
1 teaspoon dried thyme
Pinch salt
Pinch pepper
1 pound turkey cutlets
2 cups mixed greens

1. Preheat oven to 350 degrees F.

2. In a large bowl, mix mustard, lemon juice, turbino, herbs, salt, and pepper. Rub mixture onto turkey cutlets.

3. Bake for 20 minutes or until done. Serve over mixed greens.

PER SERVING
Calories 181
Calories from Fat 50
Percent Total Calories From:
Fat 27%
Protein 63%
Carbohydrates 10%
Percent RDA:
Vitamin A 42%
Vitamin C 26%
Calcium 0%
Iron 19%

Nutrient	Amount per Serving	% Daily Value
Total Fat	6 g	8%
Saturated Fat	2 g	8%
Cholesterol	69 mg	23%
Sodium	937 mg	39%
Total Carbohydrate	4 g	1%
Dietary Fiber	0 g	2%
Sugars	0 g	
Protein	28 g	

Citrus Chicken

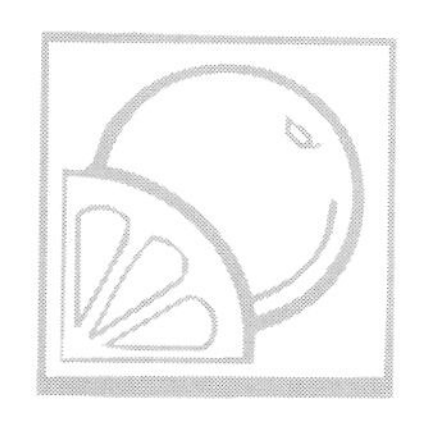

2 SERVINGS

½ cup freshly squeezed orange juice
½ cup fresh pineapple juice
⅓ cup freshly squeezed lime juice
¼ cup dry red wine
2 tablespoons Chinese dry five spice powder
¼ cup olive oil
Pinch salt
Pinch pepper
1 tablespoon chopped fresh cilantro, chopped
1 tablespoon dried thyme
2 cloves garlic, chopped
2 whole chicken breasts, boned and skinned

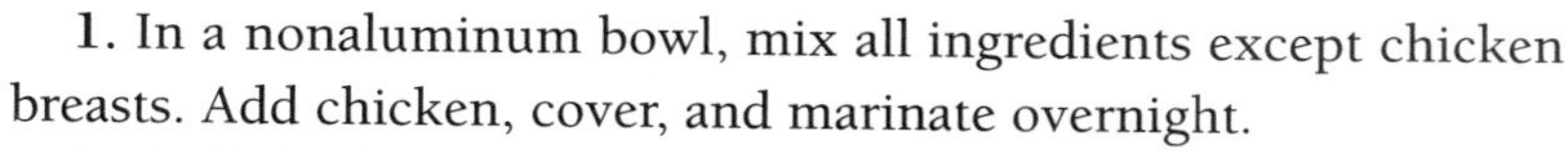

1. In a nonaluminum bowl, mix all ingredients except chicken breasts. Add chicken, cover, and marinate overnight.

2. Grill chicken over a low fire, basting occasionally with marinade until done.

PER SERVING
Calories 357
Calories from Fat 132
Percent Total Calories From:
Fat 37%
Protein 63%
Carbohydrates 0%
Percent RDA:
Vitamin A 3%
Vitamin C 0%
Calcium 0%
Iron 11%

Nutrient	Amount per Serving	% Daily Value
Total Fat	15 g	23%
Saturated Fat	4 g	21%
Cholesterol	159 mg	53%
Sodium	134 mg	6%
Total Carbohydrate	0 g	0%
Dietary Fiber	0 g	0%
Sugars	0 g	
Protein	56 g	

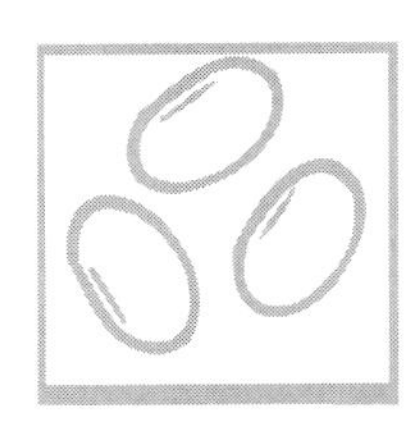

Grilled Tuna with Mango Salsa

2 SERVINGS

1 8-ounce tuna fillet, cut in half

Marinade

¾ cup orange juice
⅔ cup chopped scallion tops
⅛ teaspoon lemon zest
1 tablespoon lemon juice
½ tablespoon balsamic vinegar
2 tablespoons olive oil
Pinch salt
Pinch pepper

Salsa

1 ripe mango, diced
1 tablespoon lemon juice
¼ teaspoon peeled and chopped fresh ginger
¼ red onion, chopped
2 tablespoons chopped fresh cilantro
Pinch salt
Pinch pepper

PER SERVING
Calories 244
Calories from Fat 51
Percent Total Calories From:
Fat 21%
Protein 43%
Carbohydrates 35%
Percent RDA:
Vitamin A 124%
Vitamin C 57%
Calcium 0%
Iron 9%

Nutrient	Amount per Serving	% Daily Value
Total Fat	6 g	9%
Saturated Fat	1 g	7%
Cholesterol	42 mg	14%
Sodium	1209 mg	50%
Total Carbohydrate	22 g	7%
Dietary Fiber	1 g	5%
Sugars	0 g	
Protein	27 g	

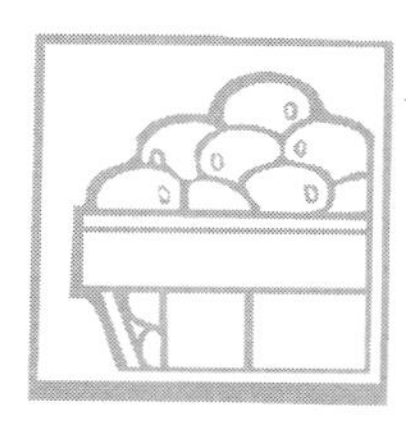

1. In a bowl, combine marinade ingredients. Marinate tuna and refrigerate for 6 hours.

2. In a small bowl, combine salsa ingredients and refrigerate for 30 minutes.

3. Grill tuna over medium heat for 3 minutes each side. Top with mango salsa.

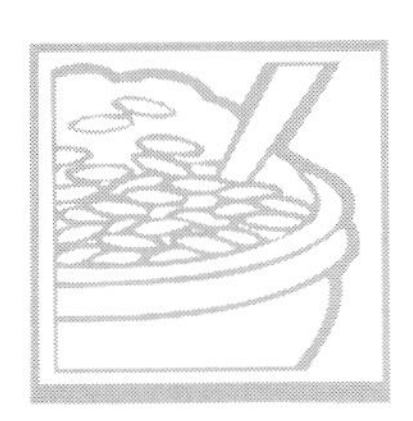

Ginger Sesame Chicken and Pasta Salad

4 SERVINGS

3 tablespoons sesame seeds
2 tablespoons olive oil
Dash hot pepper oil
Dash chili powder
2 whole chicken breasts, boned, skinned, and cut into strips
1 carrot, sliced
¼ head cabbage, shredded
⅓ cup Chinese pea pods
1 teaspoon peeled and chopped fresh ginger
1 teaspoon white vinegar
2 scallions including tops, sliced
½ cup angel hair pasta, cooked

PER SERVING
Calories 365
Calories from Fat 179
Percent Total Calories From:
Fat 49%
Protein 36%
Carbohydrates 15%
Percent RDA:
Vitamin A 106%
Vitamin C 60%
Calcium 0%
Iron 13%

Nutrient	Amount per Serving	% Daily Value
Total Fat	20 g	31%
Saturated Fat	4 g	19%
Cholesterol	91 mg	30%
Sodium	93 mg	4%
Total Carbohydrate	14 g	5%
Dietary Fiber	1 g	5%
Sugars	0 g	
Protein	33 g	

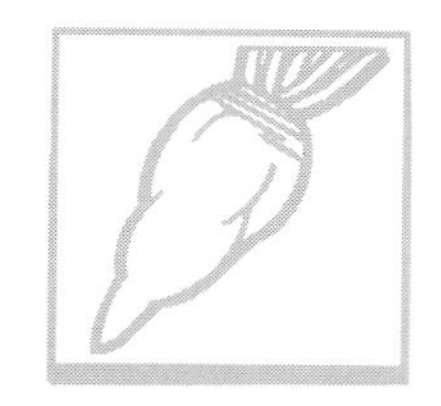

1. In a nonstick skillet, toast sesame seeds over medium heat until golden brown.

2. Add olive oil, hot pepper oil, chili powder, and chicken, and stir for 1 minute.

3. Add carrots, cabbage, pea pods, ginger, white vinegar and scallions. Cook 5 more minutes, stirring frequently.

4. Toss with pasta and serve.

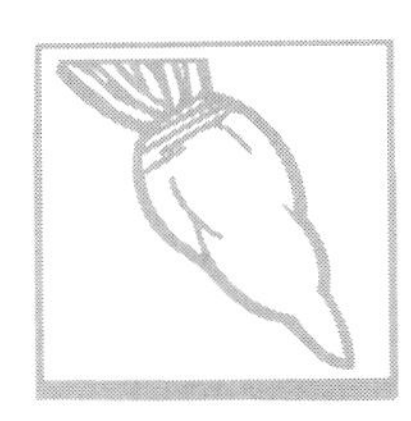

Grilled Lamb Chop with Braised Red Cabbage

4 SERVINGS

Marinade

¼ cup olive oil
1 cup finely chopped onions
2 tablespoons lemon juice
2 tablespoons minced fresh parsley
1 tablespoon chopped fresh lavender
Pinch salt
Pinch pepper

4 2-ounce lamb chops
1 red onion, sliced
½ cup red wine vinegar
1 teaspoon caraway seed
½ head red cabbage, cored and shredded
1½ tablespoons turbino
½ cup raisins
Pinch salt
Pinch pepper

PER SERVING
Calories 511
Calories from Fat 229
Percent Total Calories From:
- Fat 45%
- Protein 25%
- Carbohydrates 26%

Percent RDA:
- Vitamin A 4%
- Vitamin C 127%
- Calcium 0%
- Iron 23%

Nutrient	Amount per Serving	% Daily Value
Total Fat	25 g	39%
Saturated Fat	6 g	28%
Cholesterol	91 mg	30%
Sodium	1266 mg	53%
Total Carbohydrate	33 g	11%
Dietary Fiber	2 g	9%
Sugars	0 g	
Protein	33 g	

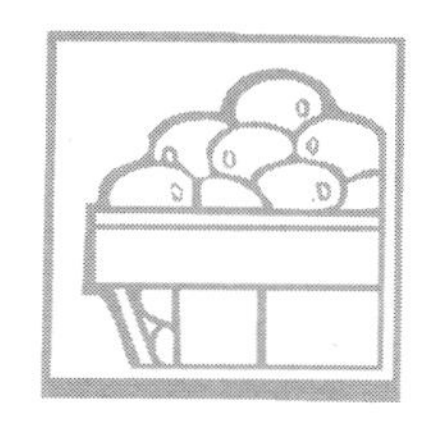

1. In a medium bowl, combine all marinade ingredients. Put lamb chops in the bowl, turn to coat, and let marinate in the refrigerator overnight.

2. In a saucepan, combine onion, vinegar, and caraway seeds. Cook until onions are wilted. Add cabbage, turbino, raisins, salt, and pepper. Cook over low heat, 20 minutes, or until cabbage is tender.

3. Grill lamb chops over medium heat, basting with marinade.

4. Serve lamb over cabbage.

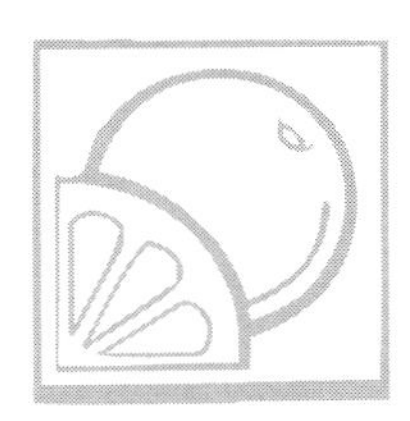

Roast Chicken Salad with Pineapple and Curry Vinaigrette

2 SERVINGS

2 whole chicken breasts, boned and skinned
Salt and pepper, to taste

Vinaigrette

½ cup lemon juice
1 teaspoon curry powder
½ teaspoon dry mustard
¼ teaspoon grated fresh ginger
3 tablespoons chopped fresh cilantro
½ tablespoon chopped garlic
¼ cup raisins
1 teaspoon olive oil
⅔ cup turbino
Pinch salt
Pinch pepper

1 head oak leaf lettuce
1 head frisee lettuce
1 head Bibb lettuce
½ cup fresh pineapple

PER SERVING
Calories 422
Calories from Fat 136
Percent Total Calories From:
Fat 32%
Protein 55%
Carbohydrates 13%
Percent RDA:
Vitamin A 16%
Vitamin C 69%
Calcium 0%
Iron 18%

Nutrient	Amount per Serving	% Daily Value
Total Fat	15 g	23%
Saturated Fat	4 g	21%
Cholesterol	159 mg	53%
Sodium	1303 mg	54%
Total Carbohydrate	14 g	5%
Dietary Fiber	1 g	3%
Sugars	0 g	
Protein	58 g	

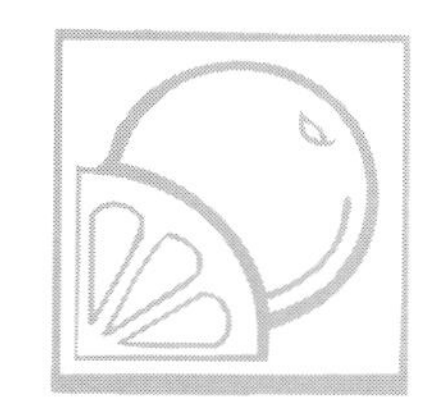

1. Preheat oven to 350 degrees F.

2. Rub chicken with salt and pepper, and bake until cooked thoroughly, about 30 minutes.

3. Remove chicken from oven and let cool. Slice cooled chicken and set aside.

4. In a small bowl, whisk lemon juice, curry powder, mustard, ginger, cilantro, garlic, raisins, olive oil, turbino, salt, and pepper together.

5. Mix lettuces, place on plate, top with sliced chicken, pour vinaigrette over salad, and garnish with pineapple.

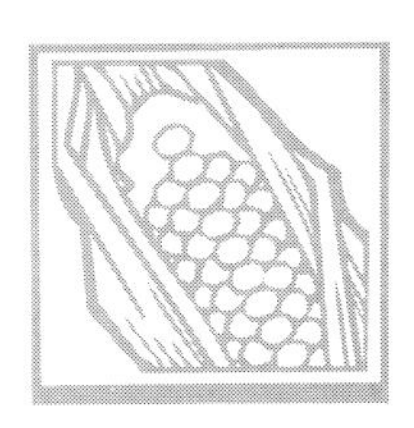

Broiled Salmon over Greens with Pumpkin Seed Vinaigrette

4 SERVINGS

Vinaigrette

½ cup apple cider
2 tablespoons canned pumpkin puree
4 tablespoons pumpkin seeds, toasted
¼ cup apple cider vinegar
¾ cup olive oil
1 tablespoon turbino
Pinch salt
Pinch pepper

1 teaspoon kosher salt
¼ teaspoon freshly ground pepper
¼ teaspoon dry mustard
8 ounces salmon fillets
2 tablespoons butter, melted
2 cups mixed salad greens

PER SERVING
Calories 614
Calories from Fat 522
Percent Total Calories From:
Fat 85%
Protein 9%
Carbohydrates 6%
Percent RDA:
Vitamin A 81%
Vitamin C 20%
Calcium 0%
Iron 8%

Nutrient	Amount per Serving	% Daily Value
Total Fat	58 g	89%
Saturated Fat	8 g	41%
Cholesterol	37 mg	12%
Sodium	1267 mg	53%
Total Carbohydrate	10 g	3%
Dietary Fiber	2 g	7%
Sugars	0 g	
Protein	13 g	

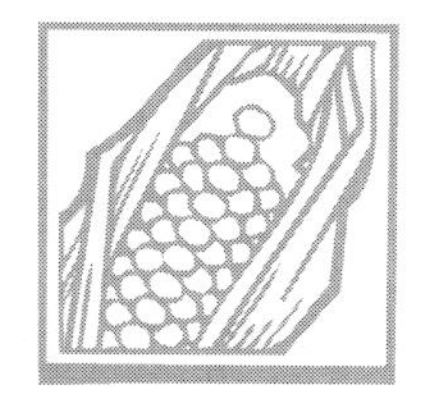

1. In a blender, combine all vinaigrette ingredients and puree. Refrigerate.

2. In a small bowl, combine salt, pepper, and mustard.

3. Brush top of salmon with butter. Sprinkle with mustard mix.

4. Broil until done, about 10 minutes or less.

5. Arrange salad greens on plate, top with salmon, and pour vinaigrette over all. Serve.

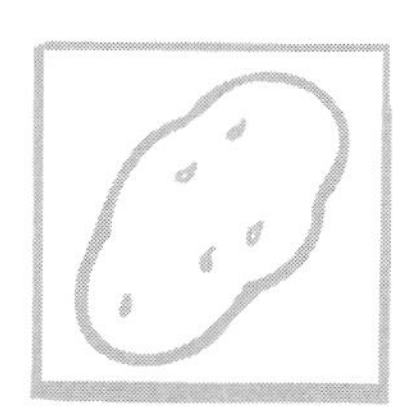

Grilled Chicken with Garlic

4 SERVINGS

Garlic Sauce

12 garlic heads
¼ cup olive oil
Pinch salt
Pinch pepper

1 chicken (a fryer), split in half
Pinch salt
Pinch pepper
⅓ cup chicken stock
3 tablespoons any chopped mixed fresh herbs

1. Preheat oven to 250 degrees F.

2. Cut tops off all garlic bulbs, exposing all the cloves. Moisten with a few drops of the olive oil and sprinkle with salt and pepper. Wrap in aluminum foil and roast in the oven for 1½ hours.

3. Squeeze garlic out of skin and puree in a food processor with remaining olive oil.

PER SERVING
Calories 159
Calories from Fat 141
Percent Total Calories From:
Fat 88%
Protein 2%
Carbohydrates 10%
Percent RDA:
Vitamin A 0%
Vitamin C 5%
Calcium 0%
Iron 3%

Nutrient	Amount per Serving	% Daily Value
Total Fat	16 g	24%
Saturated Fat	2 g	11%
Cholesterol	0 mg	0%
Sodium	1286 mg	54%
Total Carbohydrate	4 g	1%
Dietary Fiber	0 g	1%
Sugars	0 g	
Protein	1 g	

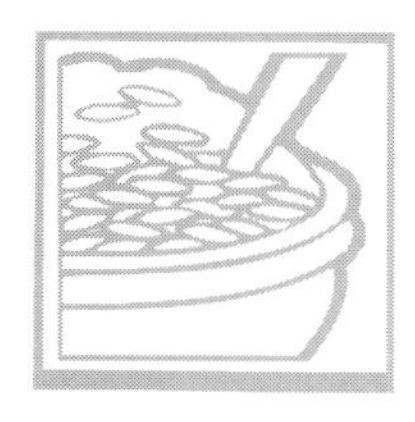

4. Rub the chicken with salt and pepper. Grill, turning once, until cooked through.

5. Raise oven temperature to 350 degrees F.

6. Place chicken in a baking dish and add chicken stock and garlic puree. Sprinkle with herbs. Bake for 15 minutes. Serve over rice.

Baked Chicken with Wild Rice

4 SERVINGS

2 whole chicken breasts, boned and skinned
¼ teaspoon ground dried sage
¼ teaspoon paprika
Pinch salt
Pinch pepper
2 tablespoons olive oil
½ onion, chopped
½ cup fresh cranberries
½ cup tart cherries, pitted
1 cup wild rice, uncooked
1 cup apple juice
1 cup chicken stock
2 pears, peeled, cored, and halved
Pinch ground cinnamon

PER SERVING
Calories 523
Calories from Fat 149
Percent Total Calories From:
Fat 28%
Protein 27%
Carbohydrates 44%
Percent RDA:
Vitamin A 5%
Vitamin C 57%
Calcium 0%
Iron 17%

Nutrient	Amount per Serving	% Daily Value
Total Fat	17 g	25%
Saturated Fat	3 g	17%
Cholesterol	79 mg	26%
Sodium	1019 mg	42%
Total Carbohydrate	58 g	19%
Dietary Fiber	3 g	10%
Sugars	0 g	
Protein	35 g	

1. Preheat oven to 350 degrees F.

2. Rub chicken breast with sage, paprika, salt, and pepper.

3. Heat oil in a large skillet over medium heat. Brown chicken on both sides and set aside.

4. Add onion, cranberries, and cherries, and cook for 2 minutes.

5. Add rice, stir, and cook for 3 minutes.

6. Transfer rice mixture to a baking dish. Add apple juice and chicken stock; place chicken on top, and add pears. Sprinkle with cinnamon. Bake for 40 minutes.

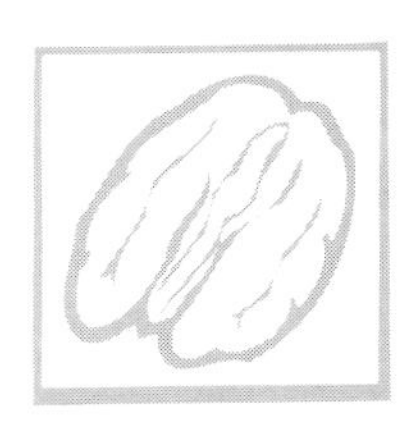

Grilled Monkfish with Spice Rub and Fruit

2 SERVINGS

1 tablespoon star anise
1 tablespoon ground ginger
1 tablespoon ground cinnamon
1 tablespoon ground cloves
1 teaspoon ground cumin
1 teaspoon ground cardamom
1 teaspoon turbino
Pinch salt
Pinch pepper
8 ounces monkfish filets
1 banana, cut lengthwise
½ pineapple, peeled and cut into rings

1. Combine spices, turbino, salt, and pepper, and warm them in a nonstick skillet for 1 to 2 minutes.

2. Rinse fish in cold water, pat dry. Rub fish with spices and let sit for 1 hour in refrigerator.

3. Grill over medium heat for 3 minutes on each side. Grill banana and pineapple and serve with fish.

PER SERVING
Calories 419
Calories from Fat 44
Percent Total Calories From:
Fat 11%
Protein 15%
Carbohydrates 74%
Percent RDA:
Vitamin A 5%
Vitamin C 133%
Calcium 0%
Iron 30%

Nutrient	Amount per Serving	% Daily Value
Total Fat	5 g	8%
Saturated Fat	1 g	4%
Cholesterol	21 mg	7%
Sodium	1196 mg	50%
Total Carbohydrate	78 g	26%
Dietary Fiber	5 g	18%
Sugars	0 g	
Protein	16 g	

Savoy Cabbage with Salmon

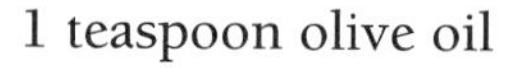

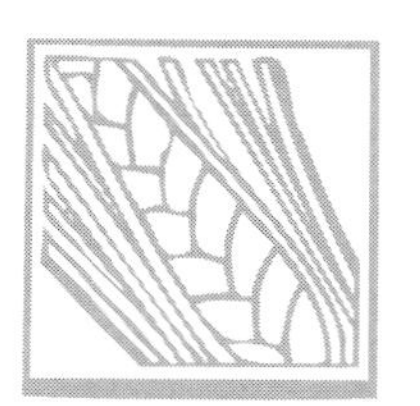

4 SERVINGS

1 teaspoon olive oil
2 shallots, sliced
4 mushrooms, sliced
2 sprigs fresh parsley
1 sprig fresh thyme
½ cup sherry vinegar
1 red bell pepper, roasted, peeled, seeded
1 cup plain nonfat yogurt
10 Savoy cabbage leaves
8 ounces smoked salmon
Pinch salt
Pinch pepper

1. In a small saucepan, heat olive oil. Add shallots, mushrooms, parsley, and thyme; stir while cooking for 2 minutes. Add vinegar and bell pepper and cook 5 minutes. Cool.

2. Pour mixture into blender and puree while adding yogurt.

3. Boil cabbage leaves in salted water for 2 to 3 minutes.

4. Place half of the leaves on a plate, top with salmon, cover with remaining leaves, and top with sauce. Salt and pepper to taste.

PER SERVING
Calories 194
Calories from Fat 55
Percent Total Calories From:
Fat 28%
Protein 35%
Carbohydrates 37%
Percent RDA:
Vitamin A 67%
Vitamin C 152%
Calcium 0%
Iron 14%

Nutrient	Amount per Serving	% Daily Value
Total Fat	6 g	9%
Saturated Fat	2 g	10%
Cholesterol	21 mg	7%
Sodium	1799 mg	75%
Total Carbohydrate	18 g	6%
Dietary Fiber	2 g	7%
Sugars	0 g	
Protein	17 g	

Crunchy Chicken with Lemon Curry Sauce

2 SERVINGS

¼ cup plain nonfat yogurt
Juice of 1 lemon
1 teaspoon curry powder
2 whole chicken breasts, skinned and split
Pinch salt and pepper
½ cup bran flakes, crushed

1. Preheat oven to 350 degrees F.
2. In a bowl, combine yogurt, lemon juice, and curry powder.
3. Season chicken with salt and pepper. Roll chicken in yogurt mixture and press into bran flakes to coat.
4. Bake in baking dish for 40 minutes.

PER SERVING
Calories 399
Calories from Fat 143
Percent Total Calories From:
Fat 36%
Protein 58%
Carbohydrate 6%
Percent RDA:
Vitamin A 5%
Vitamin C 26%
Calcium 0%
Iron 18%

Nutrient	Amount per Serving	% Daily Value
Total Fat	16 g	24%
Saturated Fat	5 g	24%
Cholesterol	162 mg	54%
Sodium	1312 mg	55%
Total Carbohydrate	6 g	2%
Dietary Fiber	1 g	2%
Sugars	0 g	
Protein	58 g	

Caramelized Salmon with Melon Sauce

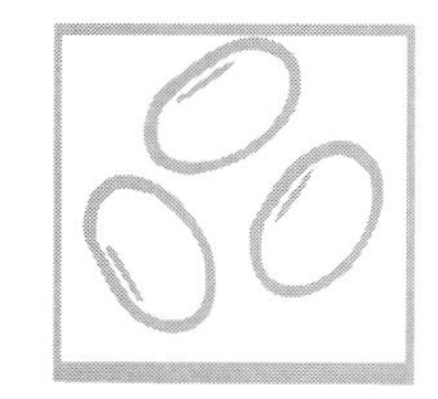

2 SERVINGS

Seasoning Rub

1 tablespoon turbino
1 teaspoon kosher salt
1 teaspoon pepper
1 teaspoon curry powder

2 4-ounce salmon filets
1 small cantaloupe, peeled, seeded, and cut into large chunks
½ teaspoon olive oil

1. In a small bowl, combine seasoning rub ingredients.
2. Rub salmon with seasoning, coating well.
3. Puree cantaloupe in blender until it is the consistency of sauce.
4. Heat oil in a nonstick sauté pan, add salmon, and cook 3 minutes per side or until done.
5. Pour melon sauce on plate and top with salmon. Serve.

PER SERVING
Calories 479
Calories from Fat 188
Percent Total Calories From:
Fat 39%
Protein 41%
Carb. 20%
Percent RDA:
Vitamin A 180%
Vitamin C 188%
Calcium 0%
Iron 12%

Nutrient	Amount per Serving	% Daily Value
Total Fat	21 g	32%
Saturated Fat	3 g	17%
Cholesterol	148 mg	49%
Sodium	1300 mg	54%
Total Carbohydrate	24 g	8%
Dietary Fiber	1 g	5%
Sugars	0 g	
Protein	49 g	

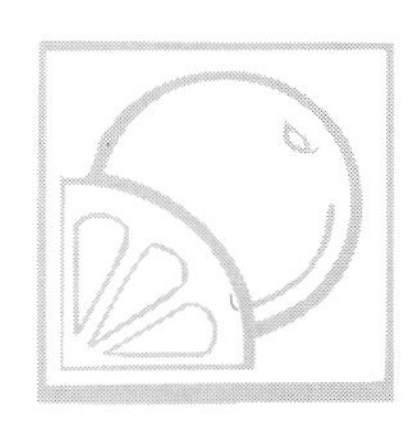

Baked Salmon with Orange Sauce

2 SERVINGS

2 6-ounce salmon fillets
Pinch salt
Pinch pepper
1 lemon, cut in half
Juice of 1 orange
Pinch saffron
1 tablespoon plain nonfat yogurt
Pinch turbino

1. Preheat oven to 350 degrees F.
2. Place salmon on aluminum foil, sprinkle with salt and pepper. Squeeze lemon over salmon and wrap in foil. Bake for about 8 minutes, or until done.
3. In a small saucepan, bring orange juice and saffron to a boil. Let cool and whisk in yogurt and sugar.
4. Pour warm sauce over salmon and serve.

PER SERVING
Calories 409
Calories from Fat 172
Percent Total Calories From:
Fat 42%
Protein 47%
Carbohydrate 11%
Percent RDA:
Vitamin A 10%
Vitamin C 58%
Calcium 0%
Iron 8%

Nutrient	Amount per Serving	% Daily Value
Total Fat	19 g	29%
Saturated Fat	3 g	17%
Cholesterol	149 mg	50%
Sodium	1281 mg	53%
Total Carbohydrate	12 g	4%
Dietary Fiber	0 g	2%
Sugars	0 g	
Protein	48 g	

Pork with Cherry Sauce over Polenta

2 SERVINGS

Pinch salt
Pinch pepper
Pinch ground ginger
1 6-ounce pork loin
1 package polenta
⅛ cup sweet vermouth
¼ cup tart cherries, pitted and chopped
¼ cup chicken stock
¼ cup cherry juice

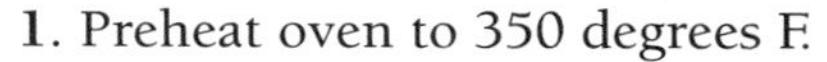

1. Preheat oven to 350 degrees F.
2. Sprinkle the salt, pepper and ginger on the pork loin. Bake in a roasting pan or ovenproof skillet for 8 to 12 minutes or until medium doneness. Remove pork loin from pan.
3. Make polenta according to instructions.
4. On top of the stove over medium heat, stir vermouth into pan drippings. Simmer until reduced by half. Add remaining ingredients and continue simmering until cherries become soft.
5. Put polenta in a serving bowl. Slice pork and arrange over the polenta. Pour cherry sauce over the pork and serve.

PER SERVING
Calories 173
Calories from Fat 62
Percent Total Calories From:
Fat 36%
Protein 44%
Carbohydrate 20%
Percent RDA:
Vitamin A 3%
Vitamin C 8%
Calcium 0%
Iron 7%

Nutrient	Amount per Serving	% Daily Value
Total Fat	7 g	11%
Saturated Fat	2 g	12%
Cholesterol	53 mg	18%
Sodium	217 mg	9%
Total Carbohydrate	9 g	3%
Dietary Fiber	0 g	1%
Sugars	0 g	
Protein	19 g	

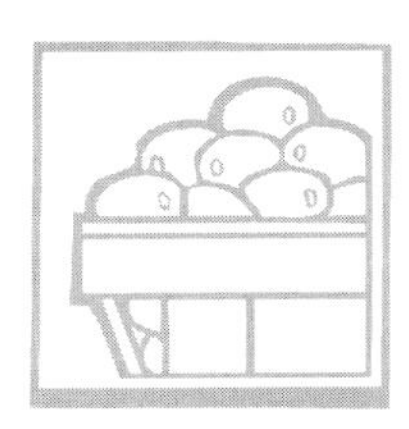

Poached Turkey with Wild Mushrooms

2 SERVINGS

Poaching Liquid

1 cup chicken stock
½ tablespoon white vinegar
3 sprigs fresh thyme
3 bay leaves
1 tablespoon black peppercorns
1 carrot, chopped
1 white onion, roughly chopped
2 stalks celery, roughly chopped

2 4-ounce turkey breasts, skinned
½ cup sliced wild mushrooms
1 tablespoon cornstarch
3 tablespoons cold water

PER SERVING
Calories 428
Calories from Fat 48
Percent Total Calories From:
Fat 11%
Protein 35%
Carbohydrate 54%
Percent RDA:
Vitamin A 232%
Vitamin C 128%
Calcium 0%
Iron 54%

Nutrient	Amount per Serving	% Daily Value
Total Fat	5 g	8%
Saturated Fat	2 g	8%
Cholesterol	63 mg	21%
Sodium	1233 mg	51%
Total Carbohydrate	58 g	19%
Dietary Fiber	10 g	40%
Sugars	0 g	
Protein	37 g	

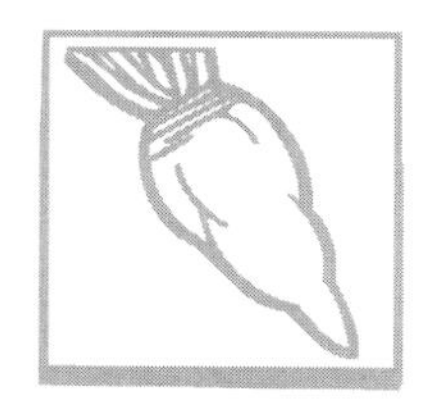

1. In a saucepan, combine chicken stock, vinegar, thyme, bay leaves, peppercorns. carrot, onion, and celery, and bring mixture to a slow simmer (slight bubbles).

2. Place turkey in liquid and cook slowly until done (15 to 20 minutes). Remove turkey, strain liquid, and pour liquid back into pan.

3. Add mushrooms to liquid and simmer until mushrooms are soft.

4. Dissolve cornstarch in cold water, add to simmering liquid, and stir until thickened.

5. Pour sauce over turkey breast and serve.

Lemon Honey Ginger Chicken

4 SERVINGS

Juice of 3 lemons
½ cup honey
1 tablespoon chopped fresh ginger
1 teaspoon salt
1 teaspoon pepper
2 chicken breasts

1. Preheat oven to 350 degrees F.

2. Mix all ingredients together, baste chicken, and bake for 30 to 45 minutes or until cooked through. Baste occasionally.

PER SERVING
Calories 165
Calories from Fat 2
Percent Total Calories From:
Fat 1%
Protein 2%
Carbohydrate 97%
Percent RDA:
Vitamin A 0%
Vitamin C 39%
Calcium 0%
Iron 4%

Nutrient	Amount per Serving	% Daily Value
Total Fat	0 g	0%
Saturated Fat	0 g	0%
Cholesterol	0 mg	0%
Sodium	585 mg	24%
Total Carbohydrate	40 g	13%
Dietary Fiber	0 g	1%
Sugars	0 g	
Protein	1 g	

Cabbage and Noodles

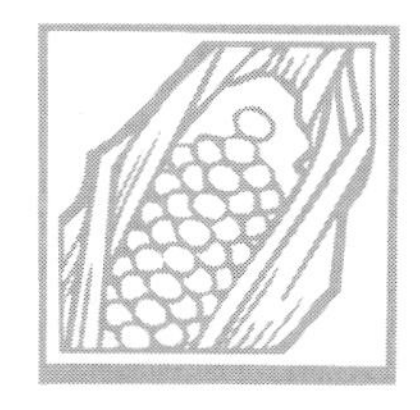

4 SERVINGS

1 cup egg noodles, uncooked
1 tablespoon olive oil
2 apples, peeled, cored, and sliced
½ head green cabbage, sliced
1 white onion, chopped
¼ cup red wine vinegar
1 tablespoon turbino
1 teaspoon caraway seed
1 cup chicken stock

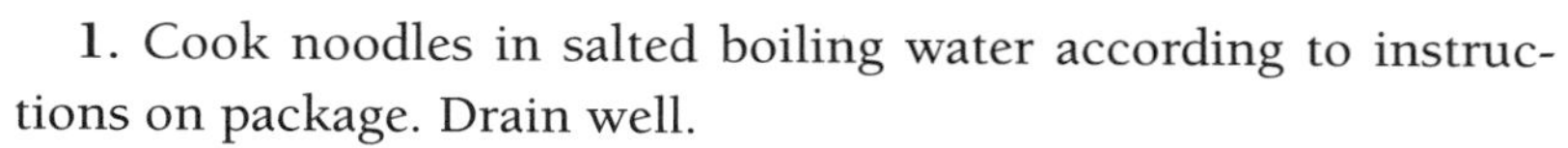

1. Cook noodles in salted boiling water according to instructions on package. Drain well.

2. In a large pot, heat the oil. When the oil is hot, stir in apples and cook until soft. Add remaining ingredients, cover, and reduce to simmer. Cook until cabbage is tender, stirring occasionally.

3. Place warm noodles on a plate and top with cabbage mixture. Garnish with applesauce, if desired, and serve.

PER SERVING
Calories 201
Calories from Fat 47
Percent Total Calories From:
- Fat 23%
- Protein 8%
- Carbohydrate 69%

Percent RDA:
- Vitamin A 4%
- Vitamin C 106%
- Calcium 0%
- Iron 8%

Nutrient	Amount per Serving	% Daily Value
Total Fat	5 g	8%
Saturated Fat	1 g	4%
Cholesterol	9 mg	3%
Sodium	389 mg	16%
Total Carbohydrate	35 g	12%
Dietary Fiber	3 g	13%
Sugars	0 g	
Protein	4 g	

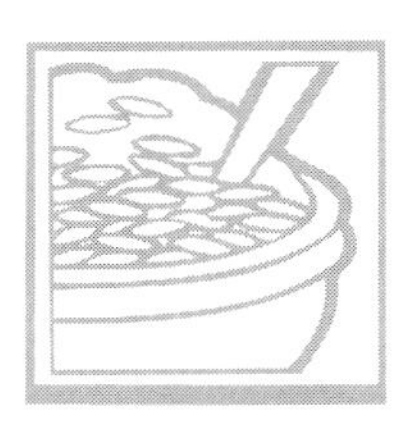

Moroccan Chicken with Rice

4 SERVINGS

1 chicken
1 teaspoon dried tarragon
1 teaspoon dried thyme
1 teaspoon salt
1 teaspoon pepper
1 cup uncooked basmati rice
2 tablespoons olive oil
½ small white onion, chopped
1½ cups chicken stock
2 tablespoons white wine
¼ cup dried fruit (raisins, dates, figs)
Pinch salt
Pinch pepper

1. Preheat oven to 350 degrees F.

2. Season chicken with tarragon, thyme, salt, and pepper, and bake for 60 to 75 minutes or until cooked through.

PER SERVING
Calories 301
Calories from Fat 78
Percent Total Calories From:
Fat 26%
Protein 6%
Carbohydrate 66%
Percent RDA:
Vitamin A 6%
Vitamin C 4%
Calcium 0%
Iron 19%

Nutrient	Amount per Serving	% Daily Value
Total Fat	9 g	13%
Saturated Fat	1 g	6%
Cholesterol	0 mg	0%
Sodium	1715 mg	71%
Total Carbohydrate	50 g	17%
Dietary Fiber	1 g	4%
Sugars	0 g	
Protein	5 g	

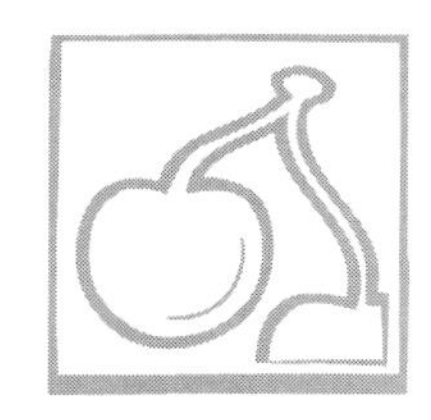

3. Rinse uncooked rice until water runs clear.

4. Heat oil in a saucepan, add onions, and cook until onions are translucent, stirring constantly. Add well-drained rice and cook for 2 minutes, stirring constantly. Add remaining ingredients, bring to a simmer, cover, and cook 12 to 15 minutes, or until all liquid is absorbed and rice is cooked.

Seared Pompano and Salsa Cruda with Polenta

2 SERVINGS

½ tablespoon olive oil
Pinch salt
Pinch pepper
2 4- to 6-ounce pompano filets

Salsa

1 large tomato, seeded and diced
½ onion, diced
¼ green onion, sliced
1 anchovy, ground
1 tablespoon chopped fresh basil
Juice of 1 lemon
Pinch salt
Pinch pepper

Polenta

1 cup stone-ground yellow cornmeal
1 teaspoon salt
3 cups cold water

PER SERVING
Calories 549
Calories from Fat 161
Percent Total Calories From:
Fat 29%
Protein 25%
Carbohydrate 46%
Percent RDA:
Vitamin A 16%
Vitamin C 58%
Calcium 0%
Iron 34%

Nutrient	Amount per Serving	% Daily Value
Total Fat	18 g	28%
Saturated Fat	5 g	25%
Cholesterol	73 mg	24%
Sodium	5316 mg	222%
Total Carbohydrate	63 g	21%
Dietary Fiber	2 g	6%
Sugars	0 g	
Protein	34 g	

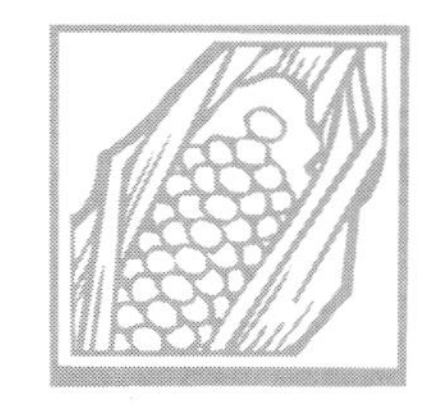

1. In a nonstick sauté pan, heat the oil. Salt and pepper the pompano filets and sear 2 minutes on each side over medium-high heat. Keep warm.

2. In a bowl, combine salsa ingredients and mix well.

3. Put cornmeal and salt in a large saucepan and gradually whisk in water until there are no lumps. Stir over moderate heat for 5 minutes. Reduce heat to low and cover for 45 minutes, stirring frequently.

4. Pour polenta onto a cutting board and spread with spatula to about a ½-inch thickness. Cut into wedges.

5. Put pompano on a plate, top with salsa, and serve with polenta.

Baked Pork Chop with Apples and Prunes

2 SERVINGS

2 6-ounce pork chops
Pinch salt
Pinch pepper
1 apple, cored, peeled, and sliced
¼ cup prunes, halved
¼ cup apple juice

1. Preheat oven to 350 degrees F.

2. Salt and pepper pork chops, place in a cast iron skillet, and bake for 8 to 10 minutes or until slightly pink in the middle. Take the chops out and set aside.

3. Heat skillet over medium heat and add remaining ingredients. Simmer until apple and prunes are soft.

4. Put the pork chops on a plate, top with apple and prune mixture, and serve.

PER SERVING
Calories 386
Calories from Fat 94
Percent Total Calories From:
Fat 24%
Protein 42%
Carbohydrate 33%
Percent RDA:
Vitamin A 9%
Vitamin C 33%
Calcium 0%
Iron 12%

Nutrient	Amount per Serving	% Daily Value
Total Fat	10 g	16%
Saturated Fat	4 g	18%
Cholesterol	102 mg	34%
Sodium	1248 mg	52%
Total Carbohydrate	32 g	11%
Dietary Fiber	3 g	10%
Sugars	0 g	
Protein	41 g	

Roast Pork Tenderloin on Mixed Greens with Pear Vinaigrette

2 SERVINGS

3 ounces pork tenderloin
¼ cup pomegranate molasses
1 tablespoon pepper
1 teaspoon chopped fresh mint
2 pears, seeded, peeled, and chopped
1 tablespoon champagne vinegar
1 cup mixed greens
½ papaya, peeled, seed, and sliced thin
½ mango, peeled, seeded, and sliced thin

1. Preheat oven to 350 degrees F.

2. Coat pork with pomegranate molasses and sprinkle with pepper. Bake about 8 minutes, or until medium (slightly pink in center).

3. In a blender, puree mint, pears, and vinegar until smooth; chill.

4. Arrange greens and fruit slices on a plate. Slice pork thin and arrange on salad. Drizzle desired amount of dressing on salad and serve.

PER SERVING
Calories 342
Calories from Fat 25
Percent Total Calories From:
Fat 7%
Protein 13%
Carbohydrate 79%
Percent RDA:
Vitamin A 86%
Vitamin C 133%
Calcium 0%
Iron 51%

Nutrient	Amount per Serving	% Daily Value
Total Fat	3 g	4%
Saturated Fat	1 g	3%
Cholesterol	25 mg	8%
Sodium	70 mg	3%
Total Carbohydrate	68 g	23%
Dietary Fiber	4 g	16%
Sugars	0 g	
Protein	11 g	

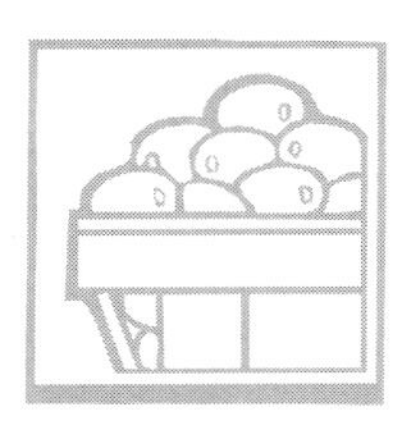

Vegetable and Pasta Bouillabaisse

6 SERVINGS

2 tablespoons olive oil
2 cloves garlic, chopped
¼ cup diced fennel
1 carrot, diced
½ small onion, diced
½ cup diced zucchini
2 bay leaves
1 teaspoon dried thyme
½ teaspoon cayenne
4 ounces monkfish filets, cut in 1½-inch cubes
4 ounces red snapper, cut in 1½-inch cubes
2 cups clam juice or fish stock
2 cups chicken stock
1 teaspoon saffron
3 teaspoons Pernod, or herbsaint
4 ounces angel hair pasta, cooked

PER SERVING
Calories 182
Calories from Fat 65
Percent Total Calories From:
Fat 36%
Protein 27%
Carbohydrate 34%
Percent RDA:
Vitamin A 75%
Vitamin C 18%
Calcium 0%
Iron 16%

Nutrient	Amount per Serving	% Daily Value
Total Fat	7 g	11%
Saturated Fat	1 g	6%
Cholesterol	46 mg	15%
Sodium	1891 mg	79%
Total Carbohydrate	16 g	5%
Dietary Fiber	1 g	2%
Sugars	0 g	
Protein	12 g	

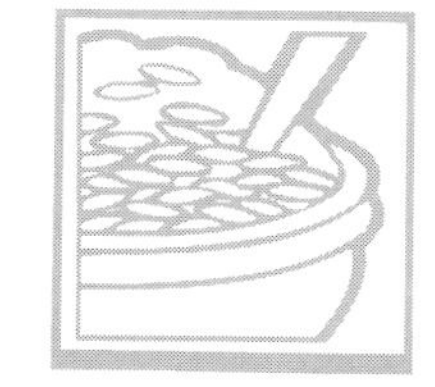

1. Heat olive oil in very large skillet. Add garlic, fennel, carrot, onion, zucchini, bay leaves, thyme, and cayenne. Cook, stirring, for 2 to 3 minutes.

2. Add fish and cook, stirring, for another 2 to 3 minutes.

3. Add clam juice, chicken stock, and saffron, and simmer for 15 to 20 minutes. Add Pernod.

4. Mound a nest of angel hair pasta in bowl and pour the fish around it. Garnish with croutons made with natural ingredient bread, a drop of olive oil, and garlic.

Spaghetti Squash with Ancho Pepper

4 SERVINGS

1 spaghetti squash, seeded and cut in half lengthwise
4 plum tomatoes, roughly chopped
1 small onion, diced
½ dried ancho chili pepper, diced
1 tablespoon chopped fresh cilantro
1 clove garlic, diced
Juice of 1 lime
1 tablespoon flaxseed oil
Pinch turbino
Pinch salt
Pinch pepper

1. To cook squash in microwave, place in microwavable bowl with ½ inch of water and bake on high for 4 to 6 minutes. Or, bake at 400 degrees F for 30 minutes or until tender. Remove flesh from skin with a fork (it will look like spaghetti strands).

2. In a blender or food processor, combine the rest of the ingredients and pulse a few times to roughly chop.

3. Place spaghetti squash on a plate and top with sauce. Garnish with fresh spring of cilantro.

PER SERVING
Calories 214
Calories from Fat 26
Percent Total Calories From:
Fat 12%
Protein 8%
Carbohydrate 79%
Percent RDA:
Vitamin A 25%
Vitamin C 72%
Calcium 0%
Iron 12%

Nutrient	Amount per Serving	% Daily Value
Total Fat	3 g	5%
Saturated Fat	1 g	3%
Cholesterol	0 mg	0%
Sodium	667 mg	28%
Total Carbohydrate	42 g	14%
Dietary Fiber	7 g	29%
Sugars	0 g	
Protein	4 g	

Ostrich with Figs and Cranberries

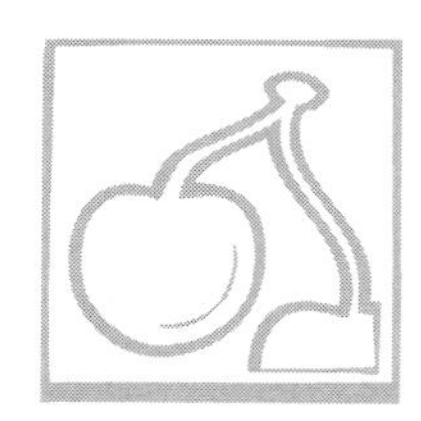

2 SERVINGS

2 4-ounce ostrich tenderloins, free range preferred
Pinch salt
Pinch pepper
2 tablespoons olive oil
1 red onion, sliced
½ cup sliced figs
¼ cup fresh cranberries, chopped
1 teaspoon chopped fresh ginger
1 teaspoon minced fresh garlic
¼ cup Madeira

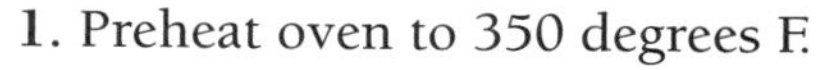

1. Preheat oven to 350 degrees F.

2. Salt and pepper ostrich. Heat 1 tablespoon of the oil in an ovenproof sauté pan and sear ostrich on both sides. Place pan in oven and roast about 20 minutes or until desired doneness. Remove tenderloins from pan and set aside.

3. Add remaining 1 tablespoon olive oil and onions to the pan and sauté until golden. Add figs, cranberries, ginger, and garlic and sauté for 2 minutes.

4. Deglaze the pan with Madeira. Reduce until sauce reaches a syrup-like consistency. Pour over ostrich and serve.

PER SERVING
Calories 241
Calories from Fat 142
Percent Total Calories From:
Fat 59%
Protein 3%
Carbohydrate 25%
Percent RDA:
Vitamin A 0%
Vitamin C 18%
Calcium 0%
Iron 5%

Nutrient	Amount per Serving	% Daily Value
Total Fat	16 g	24%
Saturated Fat	2 g	11%
Cholesterol	0 mg	0%
Sodium	1169 mg	49%
Total Carbohydrate	15 g	5%
Dietary Fiber	1 g	5%
Sugars	0 g	
Protein	2 g	

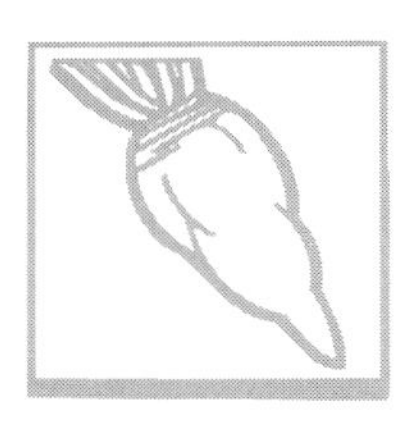

Cinnamon-seared Sea Bass

2 SERVINGS

1 tablespoon ground cinnamon
1 teaspoon ground coriander
Pinch ground cloves
4 tablespoons olive oil
1 tablespoon freshly squeezed lemon juice
2 4-ounce sea bass filets
Dash olive oil
1 apple, peeled, cored, and diced
1 banana, mashed
1 teaspoon curry powder

1. In a bowl, combine cinnamon, coriander, cloves, olive oil, and lemon juice in a bowl. Put fish in sealable freezer bag and pour in mixture. Seal and refrigerate for 1 hour.

2. Sear fillets in a nonstick skillet over medium heat for 3 minutes on each side or until done. Set aside on a plate.

3. In the same skillet, add a dash of olive oil, apple, banana, and curry powder, and stir. Cook about 5 minutes. Pour over fish and serve.

PER SERVING
Calories 414
Calories from Fat 170
Percent Total Calories From:
Fat 41%
Protein 21%
Carbohydrate 38%
Percent RDA:
Vitamin A 8%
Vitamin C 35%
Calcium 0%
Iron 20%

Nutrient	Amount per Serving	% Daily Value
Total Fat	19 g	29%
Saturated Fat	3 g	15%
Cholesterol	45 mg	15%
Sodium	81 mg	3%
Total Carbohydrate	39 g	13%
Dietary Fiber	4 g	16%
Sugars	0 g	
Protein	22 g	

Tuna Wrapped in Cabbage over Couscous

2 SERVINGS

1 4-ounce tuna fillet
Dash olive oil
Dash soy sauce
1 teaspoon minced fresh ginger
Pinch pepper
2 tablespoons chopped fresh coriander leaves
4 cabbage leaves
Dash olive oil
¼ teaspoon cumin seeds
3 dried red chili peppers
1 clove garlic, minced
½ onion, chopped
2 cups instant couscous

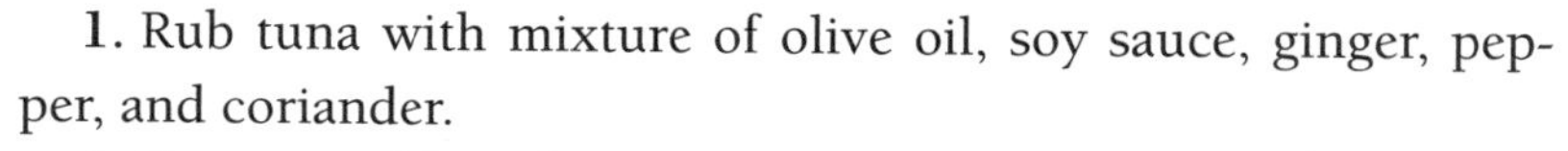

1. Rub tuna with mixture of olive oil, soy sauce, ginger, pepper, and coriander.
2. Wrap in cabbage leaves and steam for about 6 to 8 minutes.
3. In a pot, combine olive oil, cumin seeds, chilies, garlic, onion, and couscous, and cook according to directions.
4. Place tuna on a bed of couscous and serve.

PER SERVING
Calories 783
Calories from Fat 42
Percent Total Calories From:
Fat 5%
Protein 19%
Carbohydrate 76%
Percent RDA:
Vitamin A 22%
Vitamin C 6%
Calcium 0%
Iron 17%

Nutrient	Amount per Serving	% Daily Value
Total Fat	5 g	7%
Saturated Fat	1 g	5%
Cholesterol	21 mg	7%
Sodium	64 mg	3%
Total Carbohydrate	148 g	49%
Dietary Fiber	1 g	6%
Sugars	0 g	
Protein	37 g	

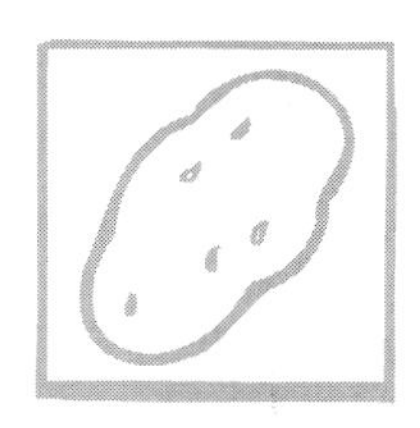

Grilled Monkfish, Fennel, and Parsnips with Honduran Cabbage

2 SERVINGS

8 ounces monkfish filets, skinned
1 fennel bulb, sliced ¼-inch thick
1 parsnip, peeled and sliced lengthwise

Marinade

¼ cup olive oil
Juice and zest of 1 lemon
1 teaspoon dried thyme
Pinch pepper

Cabbage

¼ head cabbage, sliced thin
1 tomato, chopped
Juice of 1 lemon

PER SERVING
Calories 285
Calories from Fat 25
Percent Total Calories From:
Fat 9%
Protein 29%
Carbohydrate 62%
Percent RDA:
Vitamin A 23%
Vitamin C 517%
Calcium 0%
Iron 24%

Nutrient	Amount per Serving	% Daily Value
Total Fat	3 g	4%
Saturated Fat	0 g	2%
Cholesterol	21 mg	7%
Sodium	150 mg	6%
Total Carbohydrate	44 g	15%
Dietary Fiber	6 g	24%
Sugars	0 g	
Protein	21 g	

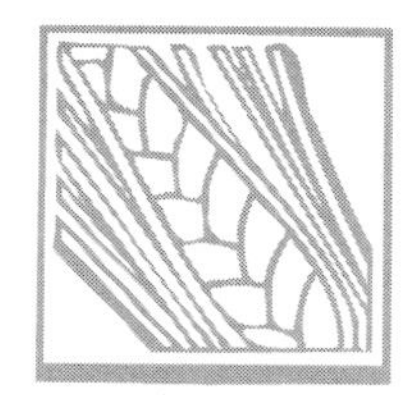

1. Place fish, fennel, and parsnips in a baking dish.

2. In a bowl, combine marinade ingredients and mix well. Pour over fish, fennel, and parsnips. Let sit for 2 hours in the refrigerator.

3. Grill fish and vegetables over medium heat.

4. Combine raw cabbage, tomato, and lemon juice on a plate. Place fish on top, arrange vegetables around fish, and serve.

Stuffed Pork Tenderloin with Fruit

4 SERVINGS

1 tablespoon olive oil
½ cup chopped white onion
¼ cup chopped dried fruit
1 tablespoon Marsala wine
⅛ cup chicken stock
½ cup bread crumbs
16 ounces pork tenderloin
Pinch salt
Pinch pepper

1. Preheat oven to 350 degrees F.

2. Heat oil in a saucepan, add onions, and cook until golden. Add dried fruit and Marsala, and cook until sauce is reduced to a syrup-like consistency. Add chicken stock, remove from heat and add enough bread crumbs to make a moist stuffing.

3. Slice pork lengthwise half-way through. Stuff with filling and tie together with butchers' string to hold stuffing inside pocket of pork. Bake 15 to 20 minutes, until medium or slightly pink in the center. Remove from pan, slice, and serve.

PER SERVING
Calories 189
Calories from Fat 60
Percent Total Calories From:
Fat 32%
Protein 30%
Carbohydrate 38%
Percent RDA:
Vitamin A 5%
Vitamin C 3%
Calcium 0%
Iron 9%

Nutrient	Amount per Serving	% Daily Value
Total Fat	7 g	10%
Saturated Fat	1 g	7%
Cholesterol	34 mg	11%
Sodium	746 mg	31%
Total Carbohydrate	18 g	6%
Dietary Fiber	1 g	2%
Sugars	0 g	
Protein	14 g	

Chapter 6

SNACKS AND DESSERTS

Reaching for the Right Stuff

DIETS AREN'T EASY. WHY? NOT BECAUSE PEOPLE GET hungry, although that is often the excuse that is given. No, it's because people are used to snacks. Yes, something to eat between meals. Maybe we do it for comfort, because it reduces anxiety, or because we're just used to snacking.

The healthy, nutritious, and delicious snacks we offer in this chapter will eliminate another roadblock on your journey to achieving improved health. So enjoy, snack away (in moderation), and be well!

Apple Crisp

10 SERVINGS

Filling

8 cups sliced tart apples
2 tablespoons turbino
½ teaspoon ground cinnamon
3 tablespoons water

Topping

¾ cup rolled oats
½ cup unbleached white flour
½ cup turbino
1 teaspoon ground cinnamon
½ teaspoon nutmeg
¼ cup canola margarine, chilled and cut into small cubes

1. Preheat oven to 375 degrees F.

2. Spread apples in a greased rectangular baking dish. Combine turbino and cinnamon and sprinkle over apples. Stir apples to coat well. Sprinkle with water.

PER SERVING
Calories 147
Calories from Fat 49
Percent Total Calories From:
Fat 33%
Protein 5%
Carbohydrate 62%
Percent RDA:
Vitamin A 5%
Vitamin C 9%
Calcium 0%
Iron 4%

Nutrient	Amount per Serving	% Daily Value
Total Fat	5 g	8%
Saturated Fat	1 g	5%
Cholesterol	0 mg	0%
Sodium	54 mg	2%
Total Carbohydrate	23 g	8%
Dietary Fiber	3 g	10%
Sugars	0 g	
Protein	2 g	

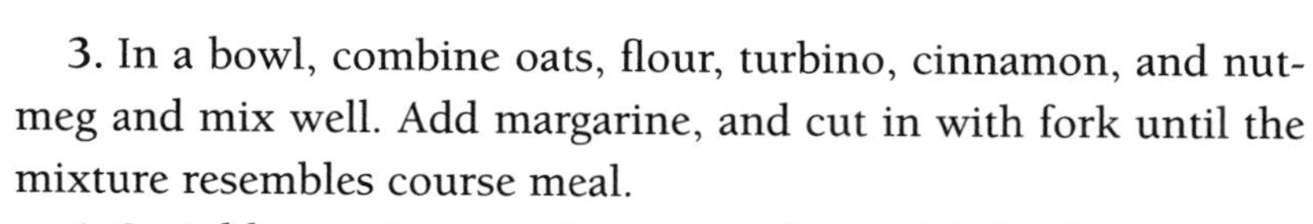

3. In a bowl, combine oats, flour, turbino, cinnamon, and nutmeg and mix well. Add margarine, and cut in with fork until the mixture resembles course meal.

4. Sprinkle topping evenly over apples and bake for 35 to 40 minutes.

5. Serve in bowls with frozen yogurt.

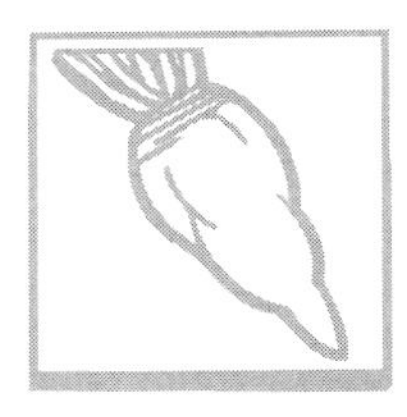

10 SERVINGS

Apricot Oatmeal Bars

1 cup rolled oats
1 cup whole wheat flour
⅔ cup turbino
¼ teaspoon salt
¼ teaspoon baking soda
¼ cup canola oil
3 tablespoons apple juice
¼ cup chopped fresh apricots and figs

1. Preheat oven to 325 degrees F.

2. In a large bowl, combine all ingredients and mix thoroughly.

3. Spread on a baking sheet and bake for 30 minutes. Let cool and cut into squares.

PER SERVING
Calories 127
Calories from Fat 55
Percent Total Calories From:
Fat 43%
Protein 8%
Carbohydrate 49%
Percent RDA:
Vitamin A 0%
Vitamin C 3%
Calcium 0%
Iron 3%

Nutrient	Amount per Serving	% Daily Value
Total Fat	6 g	9%
Saturated Fat	0 g	2%
Cholesterol	0 mg	0%
Sodium	79 mg	3%
Total Carbohydrate	16 g	5%
Dietary Fiber	1 g	4%
Sugars	0 g	
Protein	3 g	

Candied Grapefruit Peels

20 SERVINGS

3 pink grapefruits
2½ cups turbino
2 tablespoons freshly squeezed lemon juice

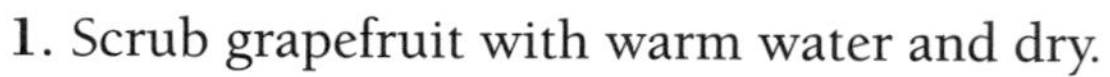

1. Scrub grapefruit with warm water and dry.
2. Peel grapefruit, with pith, into 4 equal segments (reserve flesh for another use). Cut each quarter into 6 to 8 lengthwise strips.
3. Put the peels into a saucepan and cover with cold water. Bring to a boil and blanch for 1 minute. Repeat this step 2 more times.
4. In a large saucepan, combine peels with 1 1/2 cups of the turbino and the lemon juice. Cook over low heat until almost all liquid has evaporated, 30 to 45 minutes. Let peels cool on wire rack. Spread the remaining 1 cup turbino in a shallow dish, roll each peel in it, and shake off excess. Enjoy. Use in coffee and tea.

PER SERVING
Calories 13
Calories from Fat 0
Percent Total Calories From:
- Fat 3%
- Protein 7%
- Carbohydrate 91%

Percent RDA:
- Vitamin A 2%
- Vitamin C 24%
- Calcium 0%
- Iron 0%

Nutrient	Amount per Serving	% Daily Value
Total Fat	0 g	0%
Saturated Fat	0 g	0%
Cholesterol	0 mg	0%
Sodium	0 mg	0%
Total Carbohydrate	3 g	1%
Dietary Fiber	0 g	0%
Sugars	0 g	
Protein	0 g	

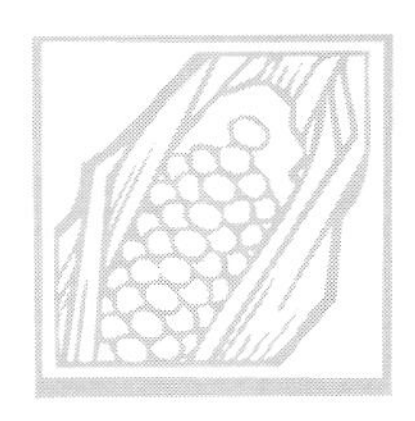

Cranberry Granola Bars

10 SERVINGS

1 cup unbleached white flour
1 teaspoon baking powder
½ teaspoon salt
1¼ cups turbino
¼ cup canola oil
3 egg whites
2 cups low-fat granola cereal with raisins
1 cup dried cranberries

1. Preheat oven to 350 degrees F.

2. In a bowl, mix flour, baking powder, and salt. In a larger bowl, beat together turbino, oil, and eggs. Add flour mixture and granola and beat until blended. Stir in dried cranberries.

3. Pour into a greased 9 × 13-inch baking pan and bake for 20 to 25 minutes. Let cool before serving.

PER SERVING
Calories 230
Calories from Fat 110
Percent Total Calories From:
Fat 48%
Protein 9%
Carbohydrate 43%
Percent RDA:
Vitamin A 0%
Vitamin C 3%
Calcium 0%
Iron 6%

Nutrient	Amount per Serving	% Daily Value
Total Fat	12 g	19%
Saturated Fat	2 g	8%
Cholesterol	0 mg	0%
Sodium	171 mg	7%
Total Carbohydrate	25 g	8%
Dietary Fiber	0 g	2%
Sugars	0 g	
Protein	5 g	

Frosted Grapes

20 SERVINGS

1½ pounds seedless red or green grapes

1. Wash grapes and pat dry. Freeze for 45 minutes. Let sit for 2 minutes before serving.

PER SERVING
Calories 25
Calories from Fat 1
Percent Total Calories From:
- Fat 4%
- Protein 3%
- Carbohydrate 92%

Percent RDA:
- Vitamin A 1%
- Vitamin C 2%
- Calcium 0%
- Iron 1%

Nutrient	Amount per Serving	% Daily Value
Total Fat	0 g	0%
Saturated Fat	0 g	0%
Cholesterol	0 mg	0%
Sodium	1 mg	0%
Total Carbohydrate	6 g	2%
Dietary Fiber	0 g	1%
Sugars	0 g	
Protein	0 g	

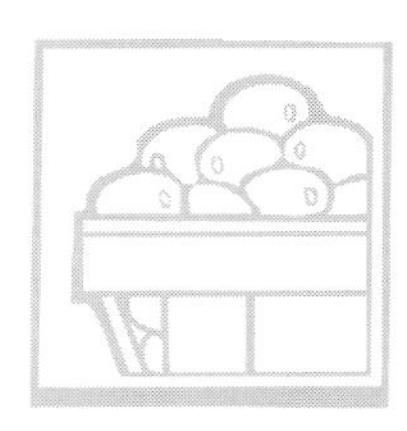

20 SERVINGS

Frozen Mixed Fruit Yogurt

3 cups mixed frozen fruit
½ cup nonfat plain yogurt
⅓ cup turbino
1 tablespoon freshly squeezed lemon juice

Sauce

3 cups sliced fresh peaches
2 tablespoons turbino
2 tablespoons brandy

1. Thaw fruit mixture to room temperature. Puree in blender with yogurt, turbino, and lemon juice.
2. Freeze for 15 to 30 minutes.
3. In a saucepan, combine sauce ingredients and heat over medium heat until mixture is warm. Serve over frozen yogurt.

PER SERVING
Calories 36
Calories from Fat 3
Percent Total Calories From:
Fat 8%
Protein 5%
Carbohydrate 77%
Percent RDA:
Vitamin A 3%
Vitamin C 6%
Calcium 0%
Iron 1%

Nutrient	Amount per Serving	% Daily Value
Total Fat	0 g	0%
Saturated Fat	0 g	1%
Cholesterol	1 mg	0%
Sodium	3 mg	0%
Total Carbohydrate	7 g	2%
Dietary Fiber	1 g	2%
Sugars	0 g	
Protein	0 g	

Fruit Compote

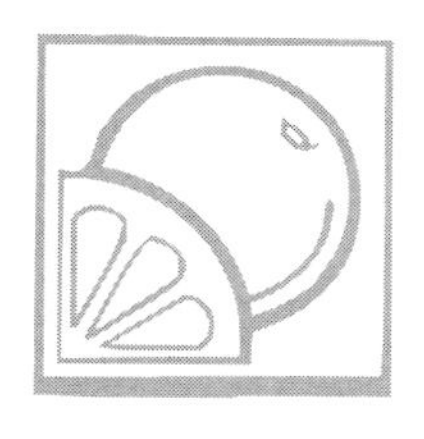

20 SERVINGS

½ pound dried apricots
¾ pound pitted prunes
½ pound dried peaches
½ cup raisins
1 lemon, quartered
½ cup turbino
1 clove
1 stick cinnamon

1. In a large saucepan, combine all ingredients with 6½ cups of water. Simmer for 1 hour.

2. Remove lemon, clove, and cinnamon stick before serving.

PER SERVING
Calories 71
Calories from Fat 2
Percent Total Calories From:
Fat 2%
Protein 5%
Carbohydrate 93%
Percent RDA:
Vitamin A 14%
Vitamin C 7%
Calcium 0%
Iron 3%

Nutrient	Amount per Serving	% Daily Value
Total Fat	0 g	0%
Saturated Fat	0 g	0%
Cholesterol	0 mg	0%
Sodium	1 mg	0%
Total Carbohydrate	17 g	6%
Dietary Fiber	1 g	2%
Sugars	0 g	
Protein	1 g	

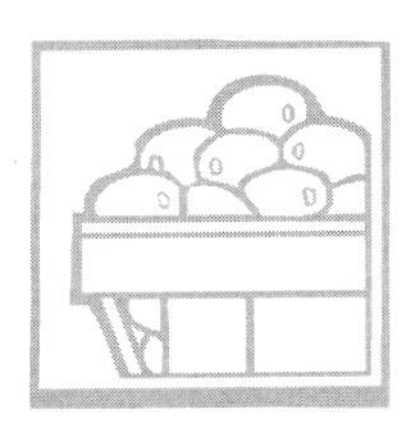

Grated Apple Cake

12 SERVINGS

- 2 egg whites
- 1 cup turbino
- 1 teaspoon canola oil
- 1 teaspoon vanilla extract
- 2 cups flour
- 2 teaspoons baking soda
- 1 teaspoon ground cinnamon
- 1 teaspoon salt
- 4 apples, cored, peeled, and grated
- 1 cup walnuts, chopped

1. Preheat oven to 350 degrees F.

2. In a large bowl, beat egg whites with turbino. Add oil and vanilla extract.

3. Sift flour with baking soda, cinnamon, and salt, and stir into egg white mixture. Fold in apples and nuts.

4. Pour into a greased 10-inch round pan and bake for 60 minutes, or until a toothpick inserted in the center comes out clean. Let cool before serving.

PER SERVING
Calories 354
Calories from Fat 224
Percent Total Calories From:
Fat 63%
Protein 5%
Carbohydrate 32%
Percent RDA:
Vitamin A 1%
Vitamin C 7%
Calcium 0%
Iron 4%

Nutrient	Amount per Serving	% Daily Value
Total Fat	25 g	38%
Saturated Fat	2 g	10%
Cholesterol	0 mg	0%
Sodium	341 mg	14%
Total Carbohydrate	28 g	9%
Dietary Fiber	2 g	8%
Sugars	0 g	
Protein	4 g	

Liquado

8 SERVINGS

½ cup freshly squeezed lime juice
1 tablespoon turbino
¼ cup fresh mint leaves
6 ice cubes

1. Puree all ingredients in a blender until smooth. Serve.

PER SERVING
Calories 11
Calories from Fat 1
Percent Total Calories From:
Fat 12%
Protein 9%
Carbohydrate 79%
Percent RDA:
Vitamin A 1%
Vitamin C 10%
Calcium 0%
Iron 3%

Nutrient	Amount per Serving	% Daily Value
Total Fat	0 g	0%
Saturated Fat	0 g	0%
Cholesterol	0 mg	0%
Sodium	2 mg	0%
Total Carbohydrate	2 g	1%
Dietary Fiber	0 g	0%
Sugars	0 g	
Protein	0 g	

Mango Lime Sorbet

10 SERVINGS

4 large mangoes, pitted, peeled, and diced
1 cup turbino
1½ cups water
¼ cup freshly squeezed lime juice

1. Puree mango in blender.

2. In a saucepan, combine turbino and water and heat, stirring, until turbino is dissolved. Cool to room temperature.

3. Add mango and lime juice, transfer mixture to a bowl, and mix well. Cover and refrigerate until chilled.

4. Freeze mixture in ice cream maker, following manufacturer's instructions. Garnish with pureed strawberries and fresh mint.

PER SERVING
Calories 62
Calories from Fat 2
Percent Total Calories From:
Fat 3%
Protein 3%
Carbohydrate 94%
Percent RDA:
Vitamin A 64%
Vitamin C 41%
Calcium 0%
Iron 1%

Nutrient	Amount per Serving	% Daily Value
Total Fat	0 g	0%
Saturated Fat	0 g	0%
Cholesterol	0 mg	0%
Sodium	2 mg	0%
Total Carbohydrate	15 g	5%
Dietary Fiber	1 g	3%
Sugars	0 g	
Protein	0 g	

Poached Apples in Wine

8 SERVINGS

2 cups dry white wine
½ cup turbino
1 vanilla bean
1 3-inch long strip lemon peel
3 black peppercorns
4 golden delicious apples, peeled, cored, and quartered

1. In a saucepan, combine wine, turbino, vanilla bean, lemon peel, and peppercorns, and bring to a boil. Reduce to gentle simmer.

2. Add apples, and continue simmering until apples are tender, about 10 minutes. Remove apples and set aside.

3. Bring mixture to simmer again and reduce to a syrup-like consistency. Strain and serve over apples.

PER SERVING
Calories 109
Calories from Fat 4
Percent Total Calories From:
Fat 3%
Protein 1%
Carbohydrate 61%
Percent RDA:
Vitamin A 1%
Vitamin C 16%
Calcium 0%
Iron 3%

Nutrient	Amount per Serving	% Daily Value
Total Fat	0 g	1%
Saturated Fat	0 g	0%
Cholesterol	0 mg	0%
Sodium	3 mg	0%
Total Carbohydrate	17 g	6%
Dietary Fiber	2 g	8%
Sugars	0 g	
Protein	0 g	

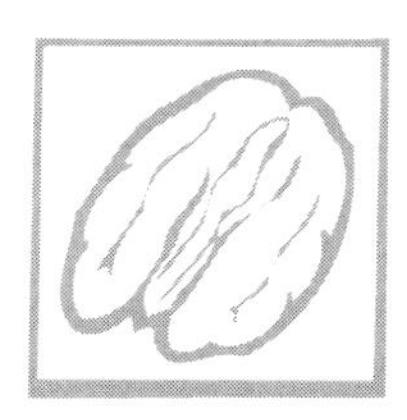

Prune Coffee Cake

12 SERVINGS

1⅓ cups pitted prunes
1¾ cups whole wheat flour, sifted
½ teaspoon baking soda
1½ teaspoons baking powder
½ teaspoon salt
¼ teaspoon ground cloves
½ teaspoon nutmeg
1½ teaspoons ground cinnamon
1 cup plus ½ tablespoon turbino
2 large egg whites
¾ cup plain nonfat yogurt
½ cup canola oil
1 teaspoon vanilla extract

1. Preheat oven to 350 degrees F.
2. In a food processor, combine ⅔ cup of the prunes and ⅓ cup hot water and pulse until smooth.
3. Chop the remaining ⅔ cup prunes and set aside.

PER SERVING
Calories 134
Calories from Fat 38
Percent Total Calories From:
Fat 29%
Protein 8%
Carbohydrate 63%
Percent RDA:
Vitamin A 6%
Vitamin C 1%
Calcium 0%
Iron 4%

Nutrient	Amount per Serving	% Daily Value
Total Fat	4 g	7%
Saturated Fat	1 g	3%
Cholesterol	1 mg	0%
Sodium	154 mg	6%
Total Carbohydrate	21 g	7%
Dietary Fiber	0 g	2%
Sugars	0 g	
Protein	3 g	

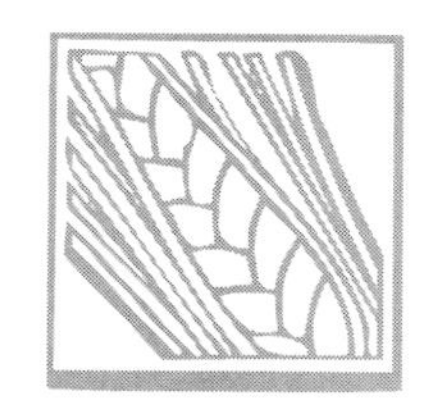

4. In a bowl, combine flour, baking soda, baking powder, salt, cloves, nutmeg, and cinnamon. In a small bowl, combine chopped prunes with 1 tablespoon of the dry ingredients.

5. In a large bowl, combine prune puree, 1 cup turbino, egg whites, yogurt, oil, and vanilla extract, and mix well. Slowly add dry ingredients, mixing on low speed. Stir in chopped prunes.

6. Pour batter into a greased 8-inch square pan and sprinkle ½-tablespoon turbino on top. Bake 30 to 45 minutes, or until toothpick inserted in center comes out clean.

Prunes and Cognac

8 SERVINGS

½ cup chopped pitted prunes
3 tablespoons Cognac
⅓ teaspoon ground cinnamon
⅓ teaspoon nutmeg
3 cups nonfat frozen yogurt
1 tablespoon chopped walnut halves

1. In a saucepan, combine prunes and Cognac. Stir over low heat until prunes are soft. Stir in cinnamon and nutmeg.

2. Put frozen yogurt in a bowl and soften to room temperature. Stir in prune mixture, freeze until firm.

3. Garnish with walnuts and serve.

PER SERVING
Calories 120
Calories from Fat 27
Percent Total Calories From:
Fat 22%
Protein 9%
Carbohydrate 64%
Percent RDA:
Vitamin A 4%
Vitamin C 1%
Calcium 0%
Iron 3%

Nutrient	Amount per Serving	% Daily Value
Total Fat	3 g	5%
Saturated Fat	1 g	4%
Cholesterol	10 mg	3%
Sodium	47 mg	2%
Total Carbohydrate	19 g	6%
Dietary Fiber	0 g	1%
Sugars	0 g	
Protein	3 g	

Rice Pudding

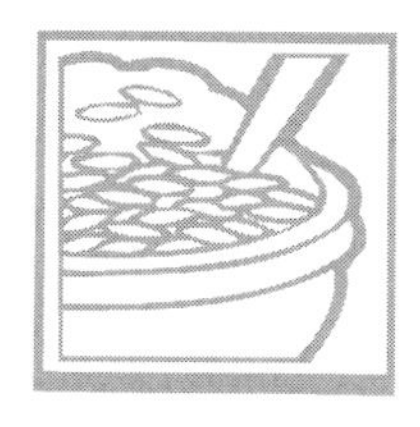

10 SERVINGS

2½ cups rice milk
¾ cup turbino
⅔ cup raw brown rice
½ cup golden raisins
2 large egg whites
1 tablespoon orange juice
1 teaspoon orange zest
1 teaspoon vanilla extract
⅓ teaspoon nutmeg

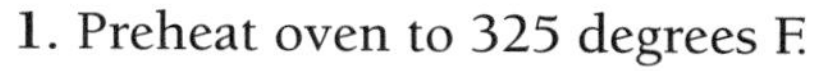

1. Preheat oven to 325 degrees F.
2. Gently bring rice milk to a boil, stirring so it does not scorch.
3. Add turbino and rice, and simmer over low heat until rice is cooked, about 40 minutes. Stir in raisins and let cool.
4. In a bowl, whisk together egg whites, orange juice, zest, vanilla extract, and nutmeg, and blend well. Stir into cooled rice.
5. Lightly coat ten 6-ounce custard cups with cooking spray. Spoon mixture into custard cups and bake 30 minutes.

PER SERVING
Calories 76
Calories from Fat 1
Percent Total Calories From:
- Fat 2%
- Protein 10%
- Carbohydrate 89%

Percent RDA:
- Vitamin A 0%
- Vitamin C 2%
- Calcium 0%
- Iron 4%

Nutrient	Amount per Serving	% Daily Value
Total Fat	0 g	0%
Saturated Fat	0 g	0%
Cholesterol	0 mg	0%
Sodium	12 mg	1%
Total Carbohydrate	17 g	6%
Dietary Fiber	0 g	1%
Sugars	0 g	
Protein	2 g	

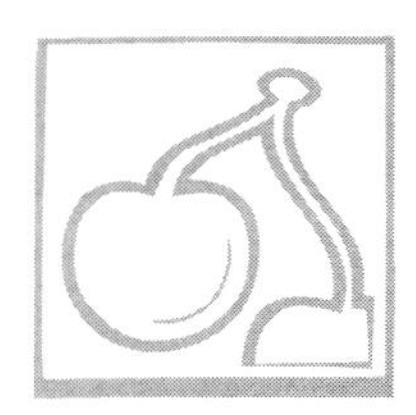

Pumpkin and Cranberry Bread

15 SERVINGS

1 cup all-purpose flour
1 cup whole wheat flour
1 cup stone-ground yellow cornmeal
2 cups turbino
1 tablespoon baking powder
2 teaspoons baking soda
2 teaspoons ground cinnamon
¼ teaspoon nutmeg
1 teaspoon ground ginger
1 teaspoon salt
1½ cups pumpkin puree, canned or fresh
1 cup plain nonfat yogurt
⅓ cup canola oil
4 egg whites
2 cups dried cranberries

PER SERVING
Calories 131
Calories from Fat 51
Percent Total Calories From:
Fat 39%
Protein 10%
Carbohydrate 51%
Percent RDA:
Vitamin A 1%
Vitamin C 4%
Calcium 0%
Iron 2%

Nutrient	Amount per Serving	% Daily Value
Total Fat	6 g	9%
Saturated Fat	1 g	4%
Cholesterol	2 mg	1%
Sodium	357 mg	15%
Total Carbohydrate	17 g	6%
Dietary Fiber	0 g	1%
Sugars	0 g	
Protein	3 g	

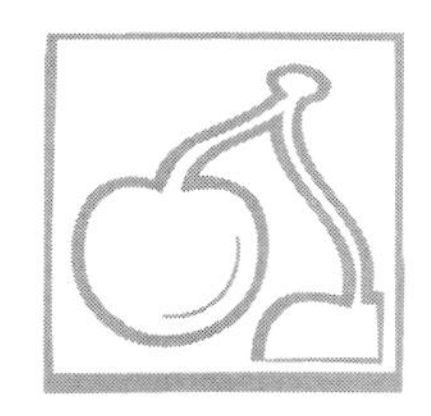

1. Preheat oven to 350 degrees F.

2. In a large bowl, combine flours, cornmeal, turbino, baking powder, baking soda, cinnamon, nutmeg, ginger, and salt and mix well.

3. In another bowl, whisk together combine pumpkin, yogurt, oil, and egg whites.

4. Stir pumpkin mixture into dry ingredients and fold in cranberries.

5. Pour batter into two 9 × 5-inch loaf pans and bake for 55 to 65 minutes, or until toothpick inserted in center comes out clean.

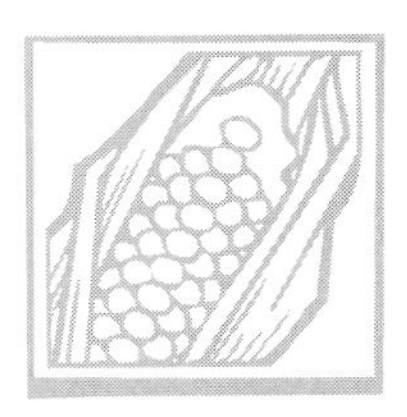

Spiced Granola and Yogurt

8 SERVINGS

4 large bananas, in peels
2 cups rolled oats
¼ cup walnut halves, chopped
¼ cup sunflower seeds
½ teaspoon ground cinnamon
1 tablespoon honey
3 slices kiwi
3 strawberries, sliced
1 cup nonfat yogurt, any flavor

1. Preheat oven to 350 degrees F.
2. Bake bananas in their peels until soft.
3. In a bowl, combine dry ingredients. Peel banana and fold in.
4. Mix honey into yogurt.
5. Place kiwi and strawberries in bottom of bowl, add yogurt, and top with banana mixture. Garnish with fresh fruit and serve.

PER SERVING
Calories 240
Calories from Fat 67
Percent Total Calories From:
Fat 28%
Protein 11%
Carbohydrate 61%
Percent RDA:
Vitamin A 3%
Vitamin C 62%
Calcium 0%
Iron 9%

Nutrient	Amount per Serving	% Daily Value
Total Fat	7 g	11%
Saturated Fat	1 g	7%
Cholesterol	4 mg	1%
Sodium	18 mg	1%
Total Carbohydrate	37 g	12%
Dietary Fiber	3 g	12%
Sugars	0 g	
Protein	7 g	

Spiced Peaches and Pears

8 SERVINGS

1 cup Rhine wine
½ cup turbino
½ vanilla bean
3 ¼-inch slices peeled fresh ginger
½ cinnamon stick
2 pears, peeled
2 peaches, peeled
1 cup raspberries
1 cup plain nonfat yogurt
3 fresh mint leaves

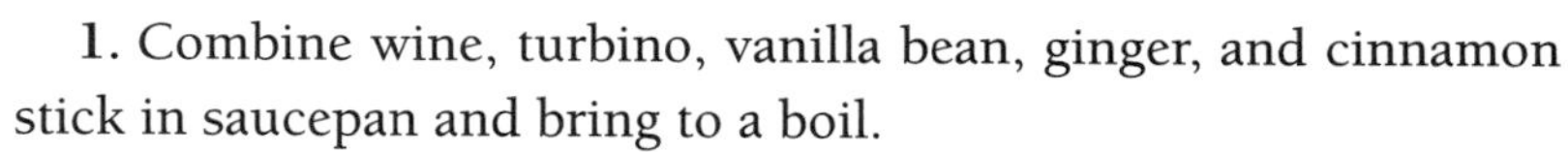

1. Combine wine, turbino, vanilla bean, ginger, and cinnamon stick in saucepan and bring to a boil.

2. Reduce heat, add pears, and cook for 5 minutes. Add peaches, and cook for 3 minutes. Remove vanilla bean.

3. Carefully fold in raspberries. Serve over yogurt, and garnish with mint.

PER SERVING
Calories 60
Calories from Fat 11
Percent Total Calories From:
Fat 19%
Protein 10%
Carbohydrate 71%
Percent RDA:
Vitamin A 4%
Vitamin C 7%
Calcium 0%
Iron 3%

Nutrient	Amount per Serving	% Daily Value
Total Fat	1 g	2%
Saturated Fat	1 g	3%
Cholesterol	4 mg	1%
Sodium	15 mg	1%
Total Carbohydrate	11 g	4%
Dietary Fiber	1 g	3%
Sugars	0 g	
Protein	1 g	

Spiced Popcorn

10 SERVINGS

1 teaspoon olive oil
1 tablespoon lime juice
⅛ teaspoon cayenne pepper
2 teaspoons salt
2 cups popped popcorn

1. Mix olive oil, lime juice, cayenne, and salt.

2. Carefully pour into large bag, immediately add popped popcorn, seal bag, and shake to coat popcorn.

3. Pour popcorn into a bowl and serve.

PER SERVING
Calories 5
Calories from Fat 5
Percent Total Calories From:
Fat 89%
Protein 1%
Carbohydrate 10%
Percent RDA:
Vitamin A 0%
Vitamin C 1%
Calcium 0%
Iron 0%

Nutrient	Amount per Serving	% Daily Value
Total Fat	1 g	1%
Saturated Fat	0 g	0%
Cholesterol	0 mg	0%
Sodium	465 mg	19%
Total Carbohydrate	0 g	0%
Dietary Fiber	0 g	0%
Sugars	0 g	
Protein	0 g	

Spiced Popcorn with Dried Fruit

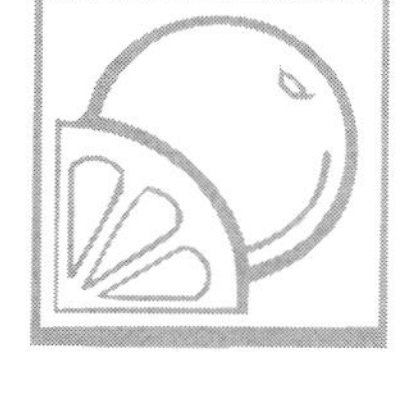

10 SERVINGS

- 2 cups popped popcorn
- 1½ ounces shredded wheat biscuits
- ¾ ounce sliced dried apples
- ¾ ounce uncooked oats
- 2 tablespoons raisins
- ¼ cup water
- 2 tablespoons turbino
- 1 tablespoon olive oil
- ¼ teaspoon ground cardamom
- ½ teaspoon vanilla extract
- ½ teaspoon salt
- ¼ teaspoon baking soda

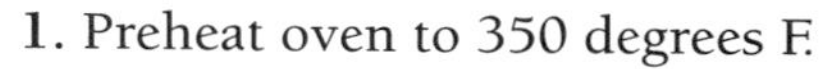

1. Preheat oven to 350 degrees F.
2. In a large bowl, combine popcorn, shredded wheat biscuits, and apples.
3. In a saucepan, combine remaining ingredients, bring to a boil, and simmer for 3 minutes. Pour over popcorn mixture.
4. Spread popcorn on a baking sheet and bake for 20 minutes.

PER SERVING
Calories 31
Calories from Fat 15
Percent Total Calories From:
- Fat 50%
- Protein 5%
- Carbohydrate 44%

Percent RDA:
- Vitamin A 0%
- Vitamin C 0%
- Calcium 0%
- Iron 1%

Nutrient	Amount per Serving	% Daily Value
Total Fat	2 g	3%
Saturated Fat	0 g	1%
Cholesterol	0 mg	0%
Sodium	137 mg	6%
Total Carbohydrate	3 g	1%
Dietary Fiber	0 g	0%
Sugars	0 g	
Protein	0 g	

Chapter 7

YOUR HOLIDAY ENTERTAINING

MOST OF US LOOK FORWARD TO THE HOLIDAYS, WHETHER it's New Year's, Easter, July 4th, or Thanksgiving, but we often tend to go overboard—we eat too much, we eat the wrong foods, and we end up paying for it. Not just with indigestion, but also with increased joint and muscle pains, fatigue, malaise, and generally feeling poorly.

Eating healthy doesn't mean eating bland food!

You can turn that cycle around with healthful and enjoyable holiday meals for you, your family, and your friends. They too can see that eating healthy doesn't mean eating bland food! We designed these tempting, tasty, appetizing, and delicious meals for two purposes: to get you rave reviews, and to keep you on your path toward a healthy lifestyle.

Eating right, eating smart, and eating healthy doesn't mean "giving up" on good taste; it means giving up the extra chemicals, additives, and preservatives that act as toxins and poisons to your body.

Eating right, eating smart, and eating healthy doesn't mean "giving up" on good taste; it means giving up the extra chemicals, additives, and preservatives that act as toxins and poisons to your body. And at holiday time, who needs that bad stuff anyway?

So invite the family, friends, or maybe even the boss. These healthy dishes were meant to be enjoyed, relished, and shared.

EASTER

Crown Roast of Lamb with
Rice Stuffing and Orange Gravy

Peach Chutney

Bouquet of Steamed Vegetables

Crown Roast of Lamb

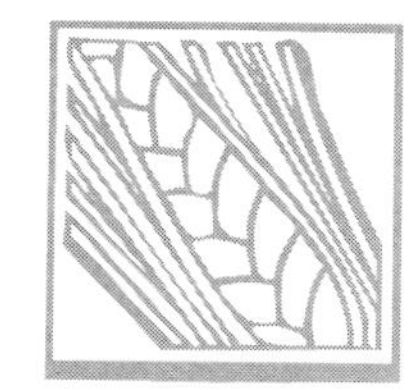

10 SERVINGS

1 5-pound crown roast of lamb, prepared by your butcher
2 tablespoons olive oil
2 tablespoons fresh rosemary
3 tablespoons chopped fresh lavender leaves
Pinch salt
Pinch pepper
Rice Stuffing (recipe on next page)

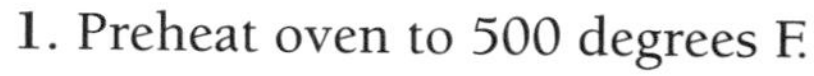

1. Preheat oven to 500 degrees F.

2. Rub lamb with oil, rosemary, lavender, salt, and pepper. Place in roasting pan with foil over exposed bones.

3. Stuff with Rice Stuffing.

4. Roast for 15 minutes, then reduce temperature to 325 degrees F. and cook about 60 to 90 minutes, or until internal temperature of lamb registers 140 degrees on an instant meat thermometer. Reserve drippings for Orange Gravy.

5. Slice and serve with Peach Chutney (page 180) and Orange Gravy (page 179).

PER SERVING
Calories 29
Calories from Fat 28
Percent Total Calories From:
Fat 98%
Protein 0%
Carbohydrate 2%
Percent RDA:
Vitamin A 0%
Vitamin C 0%
Calcium 0%
Iron 0%

Nutrient	Amount per Serving	% Daily Value
Total Fat	3 g	5%
Saturated Fat	0 g	2%
Cholesterol	0 mg	0%
Sodium	233 mg	10%
Total Carbohydrate	0 g	0%
Dietary Fiber	0 g	0%
Sugars	0 g	
Protein	0 g	

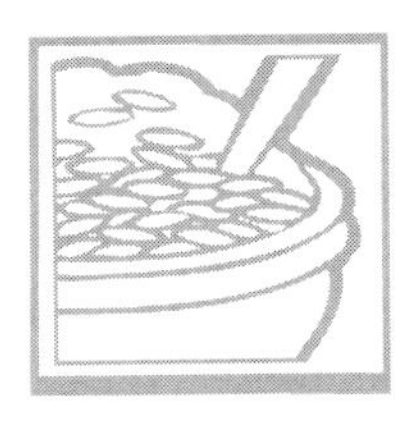

Rice Stuffing

10 SERVINGS

¼ cup shelled pistachio nuts
1 12-ounce package basmati rice, cooked
¼ cup golden raisins
Pinch salt
Pinch pepper

1. In a small saucepan, cover nuts with cold water and boil for 3 minutes. Drain.
2. In a large bowl, and combine rice, raisins, nuts, salt, and pepper. Stuff in center of crown roast, and cook as directed above.

PER SERVING
Calories 153
Calories from Fat 16
Percent Total Calories From:
Fat 10%
Protein 8%
Carbohydrate 82%
Percent RDA:
Vitamin A 0%
Vitamin C 1%
Calcium 0%
Iron 10%

Nutrient	Amount per Serving	% Daily Value
Total Fat	2 g	3%
Saturated Fat	0 g	1%
Cholesterol	0 mg	0%
Sodium	234 mg	10%
Total Carbohydrate	31 g	10%
Dietary Fiber	0 g	1%
Sugars	0 g	
Protein	3 g	

Peach Chutney

10 SERVINGS

4 peaches, pitted and peeled
½ onion, sliced
1 cinnamon stick
2 cloves
½ teaspoon nutmeg
½ teaspoon ground cardamom
1 teaspoon sliced fresh ginger
2 cups peach nectar

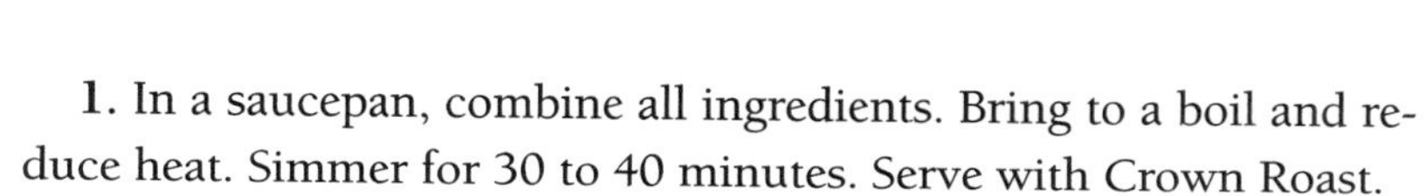

1. In a saucepan, combine all ingredients. Bring to a boil and reduce heat. Simmer for 30 to 40 minutes. Serve with Crown Roast.

PER SERVING
Calories 39
Calories from Fat 2
Percent Total Calories From:
 Fat 4%
 Protein 6%
 Carbohydrate 90%
Percent RDA:
 Vitamin A 7%
 Vitamin C 9%
 Calcium 0%
 Iron 1%

Nutrient	Amount per Serving	% Daily Value
Total Fat	0 g	0%
Saturated Fat	0 g	0%
Cholesterol	0 mg	0%
Sodium	1 mg	0%
Total Carbohydrate	9 g	3%
Dietary Fiber	1 g	2%
Sugars	0 g	
Protein	1 g	

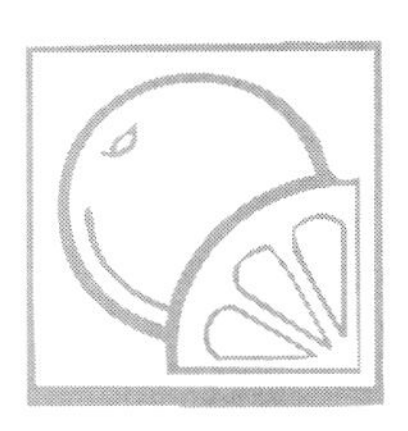

Orange Gravy

10 SERVINGS

2 tablespoons cornstarch
1 cup orange juice
1 teaspoon dried thyme
Drippings from Crown Roast of Lamb (see recipe, page 177)

1. In a small bowl, mix cornstarch with 4 tablespoons of the orange juice.
2. In a saucepan, combine reserved drippings with remaining orange juice and bring to a boil. Whisk in cornstarch mixture and thyme and simmer for 10 minutes.
3. Serve over Crown Roast of Lamb.

PER SERVING
Calories 18
Calories from Fat 1
Percent Total Calories From:
Fat 5%
Protein 5%
Carbohydrate 90%
Percent RDA:
Vitamin A 1%
Vitamin C 14%
Calcium 0%
Iron 1%

Nutrient	Amount per Serving	% Daily Value
Total Fat	0 g	0%
Saturated Fat	0 g	0%
Cholesterol	0 mg	0%
Sodium	1 mg	0%
Total Carbohydrate	4 g	1%
Dietary Fiber	0 g	0%
Sugars	0 g	
Protein	0 g	

Bouquet of Steamed Vegetables

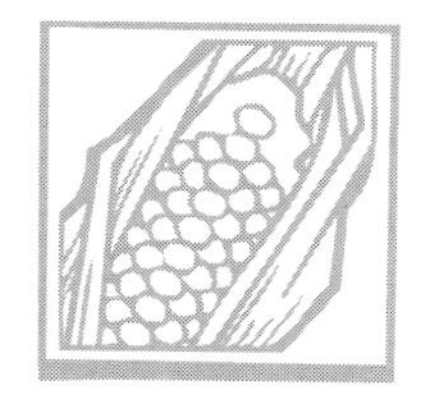

10 SERVINGS

1 head cabbage, cored and cut into wedges
12 carrots, peeled
8 asparagus spears, trimmed
1 cauliflower, trimmed into flowers
Salt and pepper, to taste

1. Combine vegetables and steam until just done.
2. Season with salt and pepper. Serve.

PER SERVING
Calories 79
Calories from Fat 4
Percent Total Calories From:
Fat 5%
Protein 15%
Carbohydrate 80%
Percent RDA:
Vitamin A 491%
Vitamin C 131%
Calcium 0%
Iron 7%

Nutrient	Amount per Serving	% Daily Value
Total Fat	0 g	1%
Saturated Fat	0 g	0%
Cholesterol	0 mg	0%
Sodium	53 mg	2%
Total Carbohydrate	16 g	5%
Dietary Fiber	2 g	8%
Sugars	0 g	
Protein	3 g	

THANKSGIVING

Thanksgiving Turkey

Cornbread and Sage Stuffing

Thanksgiving Gravy

Braised Red Cabbage

Boiled Carrots

Cranberry Relish Apple Rings

Thanksgiving Turkey

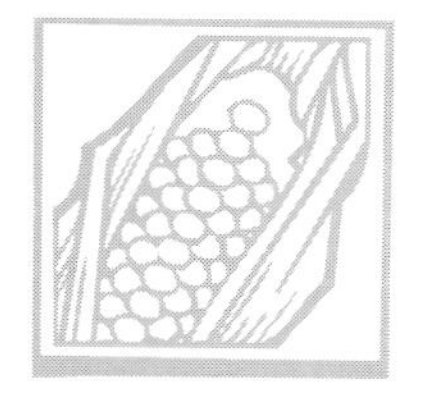

16 SERVINGS

1 16-pound turkey
Pinch salt
Pinch pepper

1. Preheat oven to 325 degrees F.

2. Remove giblets from turkey cavity. Wash turkey with cold water and pat dry. Season bird with salt and pepper inside and out.

3. Stuff loosely with Cornbread and Sage Stuffing (see recipe on next page).

4. Place turkey in roasting pan and roast about 4 hours, or until fork inserted in thigh shows the juices are clear. Baste with juices every 30 minutes. If turkey browns too much, cover with aluminum foil.

5. Remove from oven and scoop stuffing into serving bowl immediately. Carve and serve.

PER SERVING
Calories 636
Calories from Fat 279
Percent Total Calories From:
Fat 44%
Protein 56%
Carbohydrate 0%
Percent RDA:
Vitamin A 0%
Vitamin C 0%
Calcium 0%
Iron 32%

Nutrient	Amount per Serving	% Daily Value
Total Fat	31 g	48%
Saturated Fat	9 g	45%
Cholesterol	261 mg	87%
Sodium	362 mg	15%
Total Carbohydrate	0 g	0%
Dietary Fiber	0 g	0%
Sugars	0 g	
Protein	89 g	

Cornbread and Sage Stuffing

12 SERVINGS (ENOUGH FOR 14 TO 16 POUND TURKEY)

2 tablespoons olive oil
2 cups chopped onions
1½ cups chopped celery
½ cup walnut halves, chopped
5 cups yellow cornbread, crumbled
1 cup bread crumbs
1 tablespoon dried sage
2 cups chicken stock

1. Heat oil in a sauté pan and sauté onion, celery, and walnuts over medium heat until vegetables are tender. Transfer into large bowl.

2. Add remaining dry ingredients to vegetables, moisten with chicken stock, and mix lightly but well.

3. Stuff lightly into turkey cavity and cook remainder in casserole dish (or do not stuff turkey and cook in covered baking dish in 350-degree F. oven for 1 hour or until done).

PER SERVING
Calories 230
Calories from Fat 95
Percent Total Calories From:
Fat 41%
Protein 12%
Carbohydrate 47%
Percent RDA:
Vitamin A 4%
Vitamin C 6%
Calcium 0%
Iron 7%

Nutrient	Amount per Serving	% Daily Value
Total Fat	11 g	16%
Saturated Fat	2 g	9%
Cholesterol	45 mg	15%
Sodium	685 mg	29%
Total Carbohydrate	27 g	9%
Dietary Fiber	1 g	3%
Sugars	0 g	
Protein	7 g	

Thanksgiving Gravy

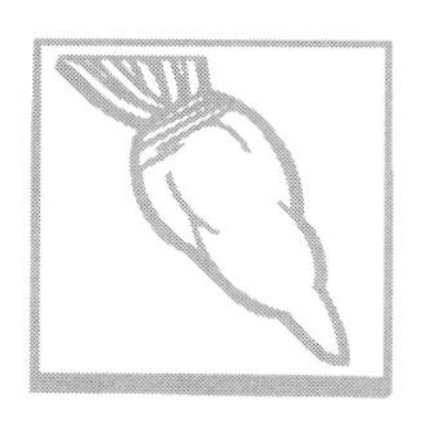

16 SERVINGS

2 tablespoons olive oil
1 turkey neck and giblets
½ cup chopped carrots
1 stalk whole celery, chopped
1 cup dry vermouth
2 cups chicken stock
3 tablespoons canola oil
¼ cup white flour
Pinch salt
Pinch pepper
Pinch dried thyme

1. Heat olive oil in a large pan and cook turkey neck, carrot, and celery over medium-high heat until brown. Transfer to saucepan, leaving the oil.

2. Bring vermouth and oil to a boil in cooking pan, and transfer to saucepan.

(continued)

PER SERVING
Calories 327
Calories from Fat 171
Percent Total Calories From:
Fat 52%
Protein 4%
Carbohydrate 24%
Percent RDA:
Vitamin A 84%
Vitamin C 29%
Calcium 0%
Iron 10%

Nutrient	Amount per Serving	% Daily Value
Total Fat	19 g	29%
Saturated Fat	2 g	10%
Cholesterol	0 mg	0%
Sodium	1519 mg	63%
Total Carbohydrate	19 g	6%
Dietary Fiber	2 g	9%
Sugars	0 g	
Protein	4 g	

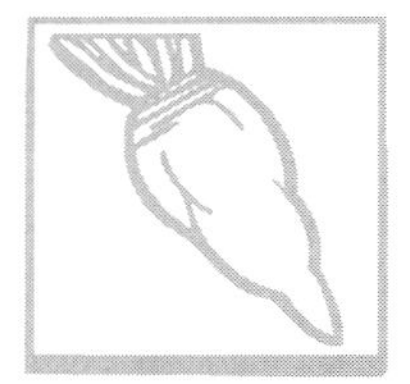

3. Add chicken stock to saucepan and simmer for 30 minutes. Strain, discarding neck and vegetables

4. Return liquid to saucepan and simmer for 5 minutes.

5. In a small bowl, mix canola oil and flour. Add to liquid, bring to a boil, reduce heat, whisk, and simmer for 10 minutes.

6. Stir in salt, pepper, and thyme, and serve with Thanksgiving Turkey.

Braised Red Cabbage

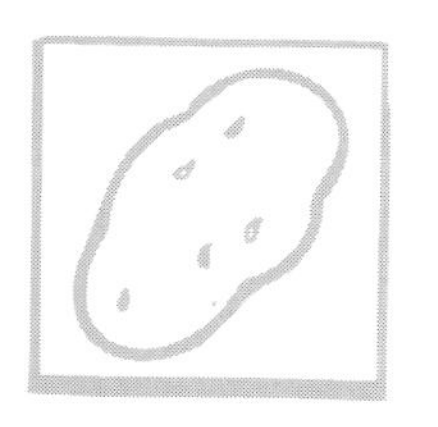

12 SERVINGS

3 tablespoons olive oil
2 cloves garlic, sliced
6 cups shredded red cabbage
1 apple, cored, peeled, and grated
¾ cup chicken broth
¾ cup red wine
1 tablespoon turbino
1 bay leaf
2 tablespoons caraway seed
Pinch salt
Pinch pepper

1. Heat olive oil in a large saucepan over medium heat. Add garlic and cook for 1 minute.

2. Add remaining ingredients, cover, and cook for 10 to 15 minutes. Remove bay leaf and serve.

PER SERVING
Calories 71
Calories from Fat 37
Percent Total Calories From:
Fat 52%
Protein 4%
Carbohydrate 31%
Percent RDA:
Vitamin A 1%
Vitamin C 35%
Calcium 0%
Iron 2%

Nutrient	Amount per Serving	% Daily Value
Total Fat	4 g	6%
Saturated Fat	1 g	3%
Cholesterol	0 mg	0%
Sodium	290 mg	12%
Total Carbohydrate	5 g	2%
Dietary Fiber	1 g	3%
Sugars	0 g	
Protein	1 g	

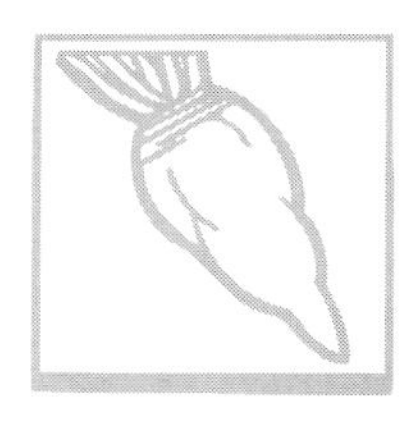

12 SERVINGS

Boiled Carrots

1 cup chicken stock
4 tablespoons turbino
1 teaspoon dried thyme
1 pound baby carrots
Pinch salt
Pinch pepper

1. In a large saucepan, combine chicken stock, turbino, and thyme, and bring to a boil.

2. Add carrots, reduce heat, and simmer for 20 minutes.

3. Season with salt and pepper. Serve.

PER SERVING
Calories 61
Calories from Fat 5
Percent Total Calories From:
Fat 8%
Protein 10%
Carbohydrate 82%
Percent RDA:
Vitamin A 640%
Vitamin C 18%
Calcium 0%
Iron 7%

Nutrient	Amount per Serving	% Daily Value
Total Fat	1 g	1%
Saturated Fat	0 g	1%
Cholesterol	0 mg	0%
Sodium	986 mg	41%
Total Carbohydrate	12 g	4%
Dietary Fiber	1 g	5%
Sugars	0 g	
Protein	2 g	

Cranberry Relish Apple Rings

12 SERVINGS

12 golden delicious apples, cored
3 pounds fresh cranberries
Zest of 3 oranges
Zest of 3 lemons
2 cups turbino
1 cup orange juice
Juice of 2 lemons
3 teaspoons grated fresh ginger

1. Preheat oven to 350 degrees F.
2. Place apples on baking sheet and bake for 20 minutes.
3. In a saucepan, combine remaining ingredients and bring to a boil. Reduce heat and simmer for 30 minutes.
4. Spoon warm mixture into apples and serve.

PER SERVING
Calories 231
Calories from Fat 10
Percent Total Calories From:
Fat 4%
Protein 3%
Carbohydrate 93%
Percent RDA:
Vitamin A 5%
Vitamin C 107%
Calcium 0%
Iron 5%

Nutrient	Amount per Serving	% Daily Value
Total Fat	1 g	2%
Saturated Fat	0 g	1%
Cholesterol	0 mg	0%
Sodium	2 mg	0%
Total Carbohydrate	53 g	18%
Dietary Fiber	6 g	23%
Sugars	0 g	
Protein	2 g	

CHRISTMAS

Steamed Roasted Goose with Gravy

Prune and Apple Garnish

Wild Rice

Beets and String Beans

Steamed Roasted Goose with Gravy

12 SERVINGS

1 9½-pound goose
Juice of 1 lemon
Pinch salt
1 carrot, chopped
1 onion, chopped
1 stalk celery, with leaves, chopped
1½ teaspoons dried thyme
1 teaspoon dried sage
2 cups red wine
1½ cups port wine
1½ tablespoons cornstarch

1. Rub the goose inside and out with lemon juice. Salt the cavity. Mix the vegetables with thyme and sage and stuff into cavity.

2. Place goose on rack in roasting pan, add 2 inches of water to bottom of pan, and bring to a boil on top of the stove. Cover, reduce heat, and steam for 1 hour.

(continued)

PER SERVING
Calories 840
Calories from Fat 487
Percent Total Calories From:
Fat 58%
Protein 30%
Carbohydrate 4%
Percent RDA:
Vitamin A 40%
Vitamin C 12%
Calcium 0%
Iron 44%

Nutrient	Amount per Serving	% Daily Value
Total Fat	54 g	83%
Saturated Fat	17 g	85%
Cholesterol	224 mg	75%
Sodium	246 mg	10%
Total Carbohydrate	8 g	3%
Dietary Fiber	1 g	3%
Sugars	0 g	
Protein	63 g	

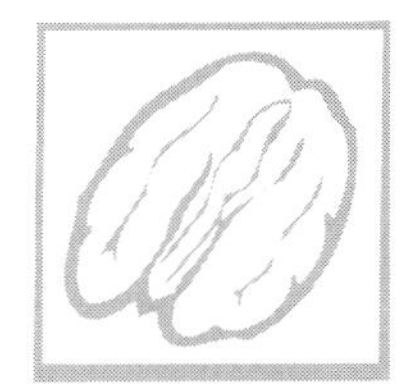

3. Remove goose from pan and let cool. Pour liquid into saucepan with vegetables from goose cavity, add 1 cup of the red wine, and simmer for 5 minutes.

4. Preheat oven to 325 degrees F.

5. Place goose on double foil-wrapped rack in roasting pan, add 1 cup of red wine, cover, and roast for 1 hour. Uncover goose and continue cooking for 30 minutes.

6. Add drippings from goose to the sauce in the saucepan. Bring to a boil, strain, and put liquid back into saucepan. Add port and cornstarch and mix to make smooth. Bring to a boil, reduce heat, and simmer for 20 minutes.

Prune and Apple Garnish

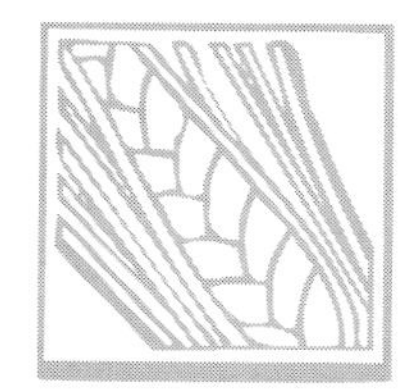

12 SERVINGS

2 pounds pitted prunes
¾ cup dry white wine
1 cup chicken stock
Pinch allspice
10 golden delicious apples, cored and sliced
⅓ cup turbino

1. In a large saucepan, combine all ingredients and cook on low heat for 40 minutes, stirring occasionally until done.

PER SERVING
Calories 387
Calories from Fat 12
Percent Total Calories From:
Fat 3%
Protein 3%
Carbohydrate 91%
Percent RDA:
Vitamin A 38%
Vitamin C 24%
Calcium 0%
Iron 15%

Nutrient	Amount per Serving	% Daily Value
Total Fat	1 g	2%
Saturated Fat	0 g	1%
Cholesterol	0 mg	0%
Sodium	151 mg	6%
Total Carbohydrate	88 g	29%
Dietary Fiber	6 g	24%
Sugars	0 g	
Protein	3 g	

Wild Rice

10 SERVINGS

1½ cups wild rice
¼ cup finely chopped mixed vegetables (onion, celery, carrot)
1 tablespoon olive oil
2 cups chicken stock

1. Wash and rinse rice, and soak in cold water for 1 hour, and drain.

2. Sauté vegetables in oil over medium heat until vegetables are soft, about 5 minutes.

3. In a saucepan, bring chicken stock and vegetables to a boil. Add rice, stir, reduce heat, cover, and simmer for 40 minutes.

PER SERVING
Calories 109
Calories from Fat 18
Percent Total Calories From:
Fat 17%
Protein 14%
Carbohydrate 69%
Percent RDA:
Vitamin A 6%
Vitamin C 0%
Calcium 0%
Iron 3%

Nutrient	Amount per Serving	% Daily Value
Total Fat	2 g	3%
Saturated Fat	0 g	2%
Cholesterol	0 mg	0%
Sodium	540 mg	22%
Total Carbohydrate	19 g	6%
Dietary Fiber	0 g	2%
Sugars	0 g	
Protein	4 g	

Beets and String Beans

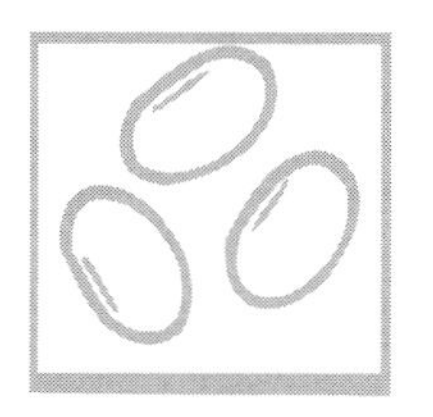

10 SERVINGS

1 teaspoon olive oil
2 pounds fresh beets, grated
1 pound string beans
½ cup chicken stock
1 teaspoon red wine vinegar

1. Heat oil in a large skillet. Add beets and cook, stirring, for 1 minute.

2. Add string beans, stock, and vinegar. Cook until beans are fork tender.

PER SERVING
Calories 67
Calories from Fat 7
Percent Total Calories From:
Fat 11%
Protein 13%
Carbohydrate 75%
Percent RDA:
Vitamin A 5%
Vitamin C 26%
Calcium 0%
Iron 7%

Nutrient	Amount per Serving	% Daily Value
Total Fat	1 g	1%
Saturated Fat	0 g	1%
Cholesterol	0 mg	0%
Sodium	140 mg	6%
Total Carbohydrate	13 g	4%
Dietary Fiber	1 g	5%
Sugars	0 g	
Protein	2 g	

ROSH HASHANAH

Vegetable Soup

Chicken in Orange Sauce

Sweet Carrots and Prunes

Vegetable Salad

Grated Apple Cake

Vegetable Soup

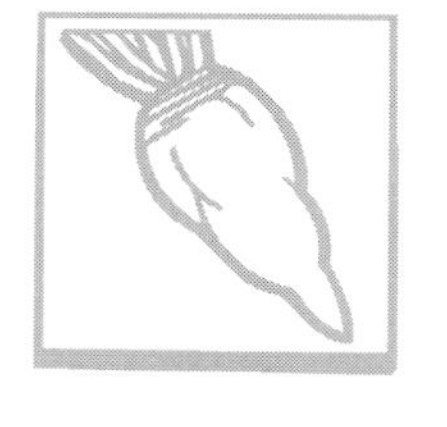

10 SERVINGS

2 tablespoons olive oil
3 carrots, peeled and sliced
1 onion, chopped
2 zucchinis, sliced
1 stalk celery, sliced
¼ cup green beans
¼ cup sliced mushrooms
6 cups chicken stock

1. Heat olive oil in a sauté pan and sauté all vegetables for 3 to 5 minutes.

2. Combine vegetables with chicken stock in a large saucepan, bring to a boil, reduce heat, and simmer for 1 hour.

PER SERVING
Calories 74
Calories from Fat 35
Percent Total Calories From:
Fat 48%
Protein 11%
Carbohydrate 42%
Percent RDA:
Vitamin A 125%
Vitamin C 14%
Calcium 0%
Iron 3%

Nutrient	Amount per Serving	% Daily Value
Total Fat	4 g	6%
Saturated Fat	1 g	3%
Cholesterol	0 mg	0%
Sodium	905 mg	38%
Total Carbohydrate	8 g	3%
Dietary Fiber	1 g	3%
Sugars	0 g	
Protein	2 g	

4 SERVINGS

Chicken in Orange Sauce

1 4-pound chicken
1½ cups orange juice
½ cup pumpkin seeds, toasted
½ cup raisins
Pinch cloves
Pinch red pepper

1. Preheat oven to 375 degrees F.

2. Place chicken in baking dish. Combine remaining ingredients and pour over chicken. Bake for 40 minutes, basting often.

PER SERVING
Calories 149
Calories from Fat 18
Percent Total Calories From:
Fat 12%
Protein 8%
Carbohydrate 80%
Percent RDA:
Vitamin A 2%
Vitamin C 57%
Calcium 0%
Iron 5%

Nutrient	Amount per Serving	% Daily Value
Total Fat	2 g	3%
Saturated Fat	0 g	2%
Cholesterol	0 mg	0%
Sodium	6 mg	0%
Total Carbohydrate	30 g	10%
Dietary Fiber	3 g	13%
Sugars	0 g	
Protein	3 g	

Sweet Carrots and Prunes

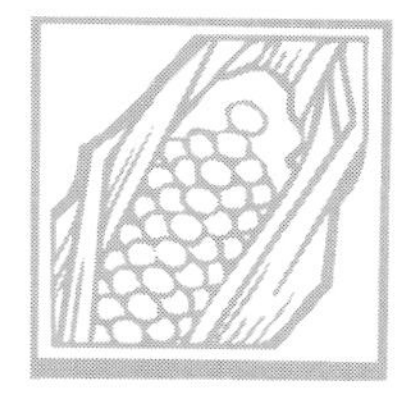

4 SERVINGS

6 carrots, sliced into 1/4-inch rounds
½ cup pitted prunes
½ cup orange juice
1 cinnamon stick
2 tablespoons turbino

1. Combine all ingredients in saucepan, bring to a boil, reduce heat, and simmer for 40 minutes.

PER SERVING
Calories 119
Calories from Fat 15
Percent Total Calories From:
Fat 3%
Protein 6%
Carbohydrate 91%
Percent RDA:
Vitamin A 68%
Vitamin C 143%
Calcium 0%
Iron 26%

Nutrient	Amount per Serving	% Daily Value
Total Fat	2 g	2%
Saturated Fat	0 g	1%
Cholesterol	0 mg	0%
Sodium	156 mg	7%
Total Carbohydrate	108 g	36%
Dietary Fiber	6 g	26%
Sugars	0 g	
Protein	8 g	

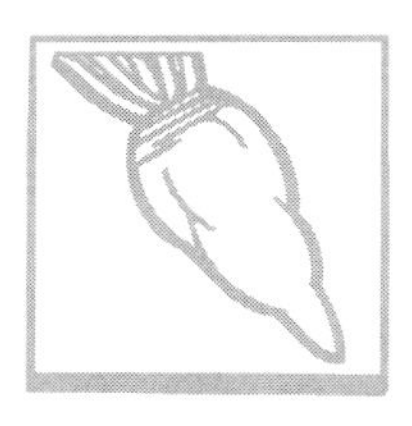

Vegetable Salad

4 SERVINGS

2 cups mixed endive, spinach, watercress, and lettuce
2 carrots, peeled and sliced lengthwise
1 beet, sliced
6 ounces garbanzo beans, cooked
1 green onion, sliced
2 radishes, sliced
4 tablespoons honey
Juice of 1 lime

1. Arrange greens on plate and top with vegetables.

2. In a small bowl, mix honey and lime juice. Pour honey-lime dressing over salad.

PER SERVING
Calories 186
Calories from Fat 12
Percent Total Calories From:
Fat 6%
Protein 11%
Carbohydrate 83%
Percent RDA:
Vitamin A 203%
Vitamin C 28%
Calcium 0%
Iron 12%

Nutrient	Amount per Serving	% Daily Value
Total Fat	1 g	2%
Saturated Fat	0 g	1%
Cholesterol	0 mg	0%
Sodium	139 mg	6%
Total Carbohydrate	38 g	13%
Dietary Fiber	2 g	8%
Sugars	0 g	
Protein	5 g	

Grated Apple Cake

12 SERVINGS

2 egg whites
1 cup turbino
1 teaspoon canola oil
1 teaspoon vanilla extract
2 cups flour
2 teaspoons baking soda
1 teaspoon salt
1 teaspoon ground cinnamon
4 apples, cored, peeled, and grated
1 cup chopped walnuts

1. Preheat oven to 350 degrees F.
2. In a large bowl, combine egg whites and turbino. Stir in oil and vanilla.
3. Sift flour with baking soda, cinnamon, and salt and add to mixture. Fold in apples and nuts.
4. Pour into a greased 10-inch round pan and bake for 60 minutes, or until a toothpick inserted in the center comes out clean. Let cool before serving.

PER SERVING
Calories 354
Calories from Fat 224
Percent Total Calories From:
Fat 63%
Protein 5%
Carbohydrate 32%
Percent RDA:
Vitamin A 1%
Vitamin C 7%
Calcium 0%
Iron 4%

Nutrient	Amount per Serving	% Daily Value
Total Fat	25 g	38%
Saturated Fat	2 g	10%
Cholesterol	0 mg	0%
Sodium	341 mg	14%
Total Carbohydrate	28 g	9%
Dietary Fiber	2 g	8%
Sugars	0 g	
Protein	4 g	

Chapter 8

ALTERNATIVE THERAPY FOR ARTHRITIS PAIN RELIEF

Vitamins, Nutrients, Supplements

WE ARE TRADITIONAL PHYSICIANS PRACTICING PAIN management, and we use standard, approved, traditional medication and therapeutic regimens for intervention. However, we are certainly not blind to the wishes and needs of our patients. Consequently, we've done some research on alternative interventions. What we have found has surprised not only our colleagues, but even some of our patients, particularly as we often recommend a combined traditional/alternative or nontraditional approach to pain management. We want your pain to go away too.

In this chapter we explore some alternative interventions. This is not an extensive or exhaustive list of supplements, nutrients, or vitamins, but a demonstration of how alternative therapies can have a role, and often a very significant role, in your overall health picture.

VITAMIN THERAPY: D AND B COMPLEX

New research reveals that supplements of some vitamins can be very effective in improving a variety of health problems, including arthritis. Here's a brief look at some of the research findings.

Initial findings from many traditional centers, including the Arthritis Center at the Boston University Medical Center, suggest that the daily recommended dietary allowance of vitamin D may be too low. Indeed, the dosage for the recommended daily allowance (RDA) is 200 International Units (IUs) of vitamin D per day. A longitudinal study over the course of eight years followed people who took this dose and people who took a double dose.

Individuals who took the recommended dose versus those who took almost twice the recommended daily allowance had a rate of osteoarthritis and joint degeneration one and a half times higher versus the people who took the double dose. So, what do we do with this information? The answer is simple: Increase your vitamin D intake.

Only a handful of foods are naturally rich in vitamin D—cod liver oil, yeast, and egg yolk. The majority of our dietary vitamin D comes from dairy products that are fortified with vitamin D, and from butter substitutes. If you live in a sunny climate, your body can convert vitamin D through your skin in response to fifteen minutes of sun exposure per day.

How does vitamin D work? We think vitamin D works by stabilizing the joints and the bones surrounding the major weight-bearing joints, thus taking some of the stress off of the joint's base, as well as off the cartilage and ligaments. Most studies on vitamin D have focused on the knee joints. These studies have revealed that there was a decrease in the loss of cartilage when individuals took large doses of vitamin D. Another theory is that vitamin D, in light of slowing cartilage degeneration, protects the cartilage itself.

The answer is simple: Increase your vitamin D intake.

Whatever the mechanism, one thing seems clear: Individuals taking less than 100 percent of the recommended daily allowance are at risk for osteoarthritis. Further, you probably need at least twice the recommended daily allowance to help slow the progression and ward off the effects of osteoarthritis.

A word of caution regarding vitamin D. This is a fat-soluble vitamin, which means it can be stored in the body. Too much vitamin D may actually cause harm, including liver and kidney dysfunction, so use caution.

B Vitamins

Two additional vitamins, sublingual B-12 and folic acid, have been shown to reduce the pain of osteoarthritis in the hands and increase handgrip strength. The University of Missouri did a small study on this issue. The dose given to study group participants was 6.4 mg of folic acid per day and 20 mcg of vitamin B-12 sublingual. The study ran for two months. On a subjective measure as well as an objective assessment of grip strength, study participants on this regimen improved more than those using nonsteroidal anti-inflammatory (Motrin-like) drugs.

There is much speculation regarding the role of B-complex, B-12, and folic acid. In theory, these B vitamins act as coenzymes or chemical co-messengers in many enzyme processes in the body, and perhaps they help to improve cartilage function by slowing the destructive or degenerative process. Nevertheless, B vitamin therapy has been shown to be effective, and should certainly be considered.

The B vitamins are not fat-soluble. Assuming that the urinary tract system (bladder and kidneys) is working well, there should be no problem in terms of taking "too much" of the B vitamins. With a healthy bladder system and excretion system, anything that the body does not need should be urinated out directly.

ANTIOXIDANTS

Antioxidants are easily obtained, readily accessible, and oh, so good for you. First of all, let us back up and discuss what antioxidants are and how and why they work.

In general, our body's chemical processes—routinely described as *metabolism*—generate what are called "free radicals." These are actually organic compounds that, by their very nature, can cause damage to tissues and to DNA, the building blocks of our body. Unchecked, an oxidation reaction occurs. This can lead to heart disease, cancer, chronic illness, fatigue, and other disease states, and to joint-inflammatory processes.

Antioxidants are a class of chemicals that can block the oxidation process. They trap the free radicals, deactivating the process of oxygen molecules, and ultimately protecting the body from this harmful cascade process.

Vitamin E

Vitamin E is so commonly available that very few people suffer from a vitamin E deficiency. It is found in vegetable oils, such as peanut and palm and sunflower oil. It is also found in many nuts, seeds, whole grains, and leafy green vegetables.

Vitamin E is another fat-soluble vitamin, so caution must be used in taking doses greater than 2,000 IUs per day. The average dose for health maintenance, arthritis prevention, and reduction of joint inflammatory process is 400 to 800 IUs per day.

Scientists don't know exactly how vitamin E works. One theory holds that it blocks the harmful oxidation process, altering the metabolism of cancer-causing agents (carcinogens) and detoxifying them so that they are unable to cause further tissue damage. Another theory says that vitamin E seems to act by accelerating cell death of damaged tissues, expediting their removal from the body. However it works, vitamin E seems to be quite helpful in the overall pattern of arthritis reduction and prevention.

Antioxidants are easily obtained, readily accessible, and oh, so good for you.

Selenium

Selenium is a mineral that has recently been shown to have relatively astonishing results. In addition to having anti-inflammatory processes, it also appears to have significant benefit in reducing the risk for various cancers, and may possibly help prevent prostate cancer and others. In the December 1996 *Journal of the American Medical Association,* epidemiologist Larry Clark showed that, in comparison to placebo, there were 63 percent fewer cases of prostate cancer, 58 percent less colon or rectal cancers, and 45 percent reduction in lung cancer.

Too good to be true? Well, it is true that in high concentrations, selenium can actually cause a toxic reaction in the body; while in low doses, selenium can be quite helpful in reducing the oxidation process and reducing the harmful breakdown products of our body's metabolism.

Selenium is found in many hard grains, and in garlic, seafood, and many dairy products. Too much selenium results in toxicity or poisoning, called *selenosis*. This condition is associated with flu-like symptoms, muscle aches, malaise, garlicky breath, and hair and nail damage. In rare cases it can lead to liver damage and respiratory failure.

As with vitamin E, we don't know exactly how selenium works. However, apparently there is some crossover with selenium and vitamin E. Animal studies revealed that rats deprived of vitamin E would die unless given doses of selenium. Apparently, one can have a crossover or masking effect of the other, inferring that there is a similar mechanism of action.

Because selenium may be toxic, discuss use of this nutrient with your family physician to make sure there are no contraindications.

While the adage "an apple a day keeps the doctor away" may be helpful for general practice, when it comes to joint pain and arthritis, it may be more correct to say that "an orange a day keeps the doctor away."

Beta-Carotene

According to the *Tufts University Health and Nutrition Letter* (September 1997), there is a possible association between foods that are high in beta-carotene and a reduced risk of arthritis, particularly rheumatoid arthritis. Rheumatoid arthritis is a form of autoimmune syndrome—the body's own immune system actively reacts to itself and the joints become inflamed. This inflammation triggers the release of a host of chemicals into the joint space and capsule, which ultimately causes additional inflammation and irritation. This causes a cascade effect and continues a spiral of inflammatory process. It appears that beta-carotene, which is an antioxidant, can fight the inflammatory process, break this downward spiral, and reduce the inflammatory reaction in the joint capsule and joint space.

Beta-carotene is abundant in various fruits and vegetables, including carrots, apricots, cantaloupes, sweet potatoes, pumpkin, and green leafy vegetables. A common-sense approach to diet, including and specifically increasing use of fruits and vegetables, is strongly recommended to obtain additional amounts of beta-carotene.

Other Antioxidants

Vitamin C is well recognized as a relatively inexpensive, simple, and safe antioxidant. It is water-soluble, which means that it is cleared by the kidney system. Assuming that the kidney system is working well, there is minimal risk. Some patients complain of mild stomach upset from increased acid; and in toxic doses it can lead to kidney stones. However, this is very rare.

Vitamin C can be obtained in capsule or tablet form, or in fresh citrus or many other vegetables. While the adage "an apple a day keeps the doctor away" may be helpful for general practice, when it comes to joint pain and arthritis, it may be more correct to say that "an orange a day keeps the doctor away."

N-acetyl-L-cysteine

A recent report by Dr. Motoyoshi Sato, MD, of Nagoya University, published in the *Journal of Rheumatology,* revealed that N-acetyl-L-cysteine can act as an antioxidant. It appears to follow the same pathways as selenium and vitamin E, leading to a reduction of the metabolic breakdown/toxic products of the body, and reducing the inflammatory-causing chemicals or toxin. Hopefully, in the near future, there will be more information on this chemical substance.

FOODS AND BOTANICAL REMEDIES

In addition to vitamins and nutrients, you may find relief in the form of botanical remedies. These are herbs, plants, and foods you eat every day.

Devil's Claw (Harpagophytom Pricumbens)

Devil's claw is a tuberous plant native to Southwest Africa. It has a vivid, claw-shaped appearance, with finger-like thorns that actually wrap themselves around the plant, protecting its seeds. Africans use the tubers, which act as underground water retainers for the plant, primarily to treat arthritis.

This natural plant has gained recognition throughout Europe for alleviating the pain of arthritis, as well as for reducing pain in general and producing an increased speed of wound healing. It is unclear exactly how the agent works. It appears to have three active anti-inflammatory ingredients that work to reduce inflammatory substances in inflamed joints, and to have substances that act to provide direct pain relief.

Africans use the tubers, which act as underground water retainers for the plant, primarily to treat arthritis.

Dr. Wallace Brawley, associated with the Biomedical Research Center in Asheville, North Carolina, has done some noncontrolled studies using devil's claw. Observational and anecdotal information suggest that devil's claw provides a significant symptom control in over 90 percent of patients using the devil's claw having improvement in pain and inflammation.

Devil's claw has no known toxicity, although it can increase stomach acid production. It should be used with great caution in individuals having peptic ulcer disease or other gastrointestinal illnesses. In addition, this is one of the agents that can be used in a synergistic fashion with additional treatments, including angelica, St. John's wort, besphania, serota, and vitamin therapy. It can be purchased in health food stores typically as a powder or caplet.

In our practice, we have made some limited use of this ingredient. Although the literature is relatively sparse for controlled studies, anecdotal studies appear promising.

Garlic

Garlic, a perennial lily, has been known for centuries in the Mediterranean region and is believed to have originated there. Garlic has long been used as a cooking ingredient, and herbalists have touted its benefits for virtually all illnesses. Recently, it has gained respect in Western medical literature as an aid to improve the circulatory, digestive, and immune systems. In addition, garlic is a relatively potent anti-inflammatory or anti-arthritic agent.

Garlic is a relatively potent anti-inflammatory or anti-arthritic agent.

As with devil's claw, we are unaware of any toxic or negative/harmful side effects. The actual dose for anti-inflammatory effect is unknown. If you don't want to eat garlic, it is available as a dietary supplement dehydrated and in a capsule, and in other forms. Begin with a low dose, such as one tablet per day, and see how it goes.

Seaweed and Sea Plants

Because human beings are composed of more than 90 percent water, it makes sense that seaweed and sea plants are an untapped source of powerful anti-inflammatory therapies. Seaweed, which is commonly eaten in Asia, has been touted as being effective in a number of arenas, most importantly as an anti-inflammatory agent.

Seaweed also has antiviral, antimicrobial, antifungal, and anticancer properties, predominantly through its immune-suppressive action. Apparently, seaweed contains a whole host of ingredients, many of which are lacking in the common Western diet. Seaweed seems to absorb nutritive elements from the ocean, and we can obtain those nutrients by eating seaweed. Seaweed has a high fiber content, many vitamins (including A, C, E, and B), and minerals (including calcium, iodine, potassium, and trace minerals).

Sea plants are an untapped source of powerful anti-inflammatory therapies.

Scientists at the National Cancer Institute in Bethesda, Maryland, are intrigued. Chemist David Neumann has studied seaweed at great length, and has found it to have amazing properties, particularly untapped properties for cancer reduction. Seaweed apparently acts like an antioxidant. Indeed it apparently has some role in detoxifying the body, almost performing a natural or fiber chelation of harmful ingredients from the body.

In iodine-sensitive individuals, seaweed may cause acne to flare up or other dermatologic reactions. Avoid seaweed if you or your physician have noted any iodine-based sensitivities.

The Good Fats: Omega-3 Fatty Acids

After years of trying to eliminate essentially all fats from the American diet, researchers are now finding out that if we want to reduce heart disease, stroke, arthritis, and hypertension, as well as reduce the risks for some types of cancers, then *adding* a little fat may be the answer!

Not all fat is bad fat. Some fats can actually help: by protecting blood vessel walls, reducing inflammatory reaction, protecting against free radicals and oxidant breakdown products, and increasing or bolstering the body's immune system.

What is this miracle ingredient? It is omega 3 fats, found in fish and a number of other foods. According to the National Fisheries Institute, salmon, sardines, shark, trout, and tuna seem to have the highest content of omega 3 fats per 3½-ounce serving. Other sources include spinach, mustard greens, wheat germ, walnuts, flaxseed, tofu, soybean oil, and canola oil. However, these ingredients need to be converted, and are approximately one-tenth as efficient as a direct intake of omega 3 oils from fresh seafood.

But a word of caution: Omega 3's activity thins the blood, reducing the risks for blood clotting. But it may also accelerate bleeding, placing people who are at high risk for hemorrhage and bleeding strokes, as well as bleeding disorders, at risk. Individuals taking aspirin, vitamin E, or anti-clotting agents should discuss this with their physician, and consider avoiding this dangerous interaction.

The bottom line? When it comes to omega 3s, eat your fish. It's no longer just brain food, but total body food.

After years of trying to eliminate essentially all fats from the American diet, researchers are now finding out that if we want to reduce heart disease, stroke, arthritis, and hypertension, as well as reduce the risks for some types of cancers, then adding *a little fat may be the answer!*

Turmeric: An Ancient Spice with New Applications

Turmeric is an ancient spice that dates back to the time of the Egyptian pharaohs. It is very similar to ginger, and is most often used in the dried, powdered form found in the spice section of your market.

Turmeric is a common ingredient in curries, and is used both as a spice and a remedy by almost all Asian cultures. It has been

The bottom line? When it comes to omega 3s, eat your fish. It's no longer just brain food, but total body food.

considered a medicine for over 5,000 years, particularly in Ayurvedic medicine. Traditionally considered an herbal equivalent of aspirin and cortisone, turmeric has been used to reduce swelling from bruises and wounds and to reduce inflammation from insect bites. Western medicine is only now beginning to understand the role of turmeric as an anti-inflammatory, anticancer, and antioxidant agent.

As we age, the body becomes less able to detoxify free radicals and less effective at managing the body's breakdown or metabolic waste products. This decreased capability, combined with decreased physical activity and altered or poor nutrition (common problems in older individuals), contribute to an overall decline of the body's immune and detoxification process. Turmeric seems to augment the body's immune system, particularly in the fight against breakdown products. How does it work? It may act by directly stimulating release of additional adrenal gland chemicals called *corticosteroids*, the body's natural cortisone. Turmeric may also work by preventing the breakdown of cortisol, allowing the cortisone in the body to act for longer periods of time.

Turmeric is a common ingredient in curries, and is used both as a spice and a remedy by almost all Asian cultures.

Unlike synthetic cortisone products and nonsteroidal anti-inflammatory agents, turmeric seems to have no toxic side effects. In fact, turmeric has been rated by the editors of Time Life Books in *The Alternative Advisor* (1997) as one of the seventy-five most effective herbs. Michael Murray, ND, a teacher of natural medicine at Bastyr University in Washington, feels that generous doses of turmeric seem to increase its full medicinal effects. Recommended dosage is 250 mg to 500 mg three times a day. Apparently, this is one spice that is no longer relegated just to the kitchen, but also appears right at home in the medicine cabinet.

Dan Shen

It is beyond the scope of this text to go into great detail discussing the concept of traditional Chinese medicine, Chinese tonics, and herbal tonic therapies. However, one herb, *dan shen*, also called purple sage or red-rooted sage, is an herb that has been traditionally used in the treatment of arthritis.

Apparently, dan shen plays a key role in circulation, increasing the body's fluid flow and acting as an immune-boosting agent. As with some other natural ingredients that improve arthritis, dan shen can aggravate a bleeding disorder. Therefore, use of this tonic in combination with vitamin E, anti-platelet therapy, or blood-thinning therapy such as Coumadin, is to be performed cautiously. Consult your physician.

Apparently, dan shen plays a key role in circulation, increasing the body's fluid flow and acting as an immune-boosting agent.

Almonds, the Healthy Nuts

Dieters, especially those interested in lowering cholesterol and reducing fat, have been warned to avoid nuts due to the high calorie contents. But what we believed fifteen, ten, and even five years ago may not be entirely accurate. The jury is still out on almonds, and clearly more research needs to be performed. But what we are learning is intriguing.

While it is true that almonds are high in calories, it is also true that they are a rich source of mono-unsaturated fats and vitamin E, and are a very good source of riboflavin, calcium, copper, and magnesium. In addition, almonds contain many natural phytochemicals, which can act as antioxidants. They can also increase circulation, reduce cardiac disease, and—most important—reduce inflammation and painful swollen arthritic joints. Benzaldehyde, a key anti-inflammatory ingredient in almonds, apparently has strong/potent anti-inflammatory effects.

Dieters, especially those interested in lowering cholesterol and reducing fat, have been warned to avoid nuts due to the high calorie contents; however, the jury is still out on almonds.

St. John's Wort

St. John's wort, or hypericum, is an herb and one of the most popular antidepressants in Germany, outselling Prozac 7 to 1 in one recent study. Interestingly, while there has been much written about St. John's wort for its antidepressant effect, very little has been written on its role in lifting depression from people with chronic pain.

Many arthritis sufferers have *occult depression,* a result of chronic pain. Chronic joint pain and muscle inflammation from arthritis is like a dripping water faucet—one day of a dripping faucet is simply annoying, but week after week it becomes torture. Clearly, living with constant pain can be depressing.

Research has revealed that St. John's wort can be quite effective in relieving depression. It is relatively inexpensive, and may be worthwhile to include this in the overall complement of therapeutic regimen for treating a patient for his chronic arthritis pain leading to occult depression. Dosage is 2 to 4 gm of St. John's wort extract per day.

A number of our patients taking St. John's wort have claimed significant reduction in their symptoms of pain and depression.

A number of our patients taking St. John's wort have claimed significant reduction in their symptoms of pain and depression. More important, their rating of pain has dropped significantly. We recommend this simple ingredient to our patients.

VALERIAN

Another adjunct therapy in the treatment of arthritis is sleep therapy—getting enough sleep is vital to your overall health a sense of well-being. Melatonin has enjoyed the spotlight recently in this regard, even making the cover of *Time* magazine; but we feel that melatonin needs to be used with some caution. There are some side effects, and although it seems to be relatively safe, it does need to be monitored.

However, we do find that valerian, a herb used to treat multiple ills since the first century, is quite effective for initiating sleep. In one placebo-controlled trial, 89 percent of individuals reported improved sleep, while 44 percent reported "perfect sleep."

Valerian is frequently used in Europe help to break addictions, particularly to Valium-type sleep medications. The Commission on Nutrient and Vitamin Therapy recommends 2 to 3 gm of the powdered fruit or extract, and up to 1 teaspoon of the tincture taken before bedtime. It can be quite helpful in the therapeutic regimen for overall treatment of arthritis, arthritis pain relief, and sleep initiation associated with chronic arthritis pain.

THE BOTTOM LINE

This chapter has demonstrated that many natural remedies may be quite successful in bringing relief from arthritis pain. Please don't follow the adage "Don't ask, don't tell" when it comes to trying natural substances or alternative therapies for your arthritis pain relief. There are many new and relatively exciting discoveries, and more are being made every day. Even the most traditional of physicians is now becoming aware of the utility and value of alternative therapies.

Discuss them with your physician as treatment options in addition to your regular pain medication. Do your homework, do your research, but most of all keep open communication between you and your physician. Using a combined approach, of diet, exercise, alternative therapeutic regimen, and a healthy lifestyle, you may be able to improve your arthritis syndrome significantly, and even achieve near-complete arthritis relief.

Chapter 9

A TALE OF TWO SUPPLEMENTS

Glucosamine Sulfate and Chondroitin Sulfate

GLUCOSAMINE SULFATE AND CHONDROITIN SULFATE ARE natural ingredients touted as a "miracle cure" in the book *The Arthritis Cure* by Jason Theodosakis, MD, and are currently receiving a lot of attention from physicians and patients alike. Research continues, but this chapter centers on what we have learned about these two substances, based on our own clinical experience, multiple anecdotal stories from patients, and additional research.

WE ALL WANT AN INSTANT CURE

We are two board-certified neurologists who spend a great deal of time dealing with our subspecialty of pain management. As pain goes on longer and longer unabated, it becomes suffering, taking over every aspect of our patients' lives. We know that when people hurt, they want that pain controlled. If it can't be gone altogether (everyone's first choice!), then they want it diminished to a lower and more tolerable level.

In our twenty-five years of combined practice, we've seen many approaches to pain management. What works for one person may not help at all for another. Yet, if a treatment option provides the "option" of pain management and does not have a significant risk or side effect, certainly it should be considered. In this context, glucosamine sulfate and chondroitin sulfate are two substances that have recently been used, with some success, for the treatment of chronic osteoarthritis pain.

WHAT IS GLUCOSAMINE SULFATE?

Glucosamine sulfate is a naturally occurring substance found in large concentrations in healthy animal joints. It appears to increase cartilage components. What is it comprised of? A key element is inside the cartilage meshwork of a joint: the chondrocyte, the only true cellular component in the meshwork. The chondrocyte is itself a primary source of two components in the mesh work: collagen and proteoglycans.

Think of a fish net with tightly woven mesh. The cartilage meshwork forms the cross-links of collagen in the net. The proteoglycans are fluid-loving substances that give the cartilage its spongy, resilient, shock absorber qualities that help to cushion the impact that is transmitted throughout bodies and joints with each and every activity that we perform.

WHAT HAPPENS WHEN YOU MOVE YOUR JOINTS?

When you use a joint, your action causes both compression and relaxation of the cartilage. This is very important because the cartilage is "vascular," which means that it doesn't have a direct blood supply. Cartilage receives fluids, nutrition, inflow of cartilage, and joint-building substances through diffusion from the synovial fluid, the fluid in the joint space. It's very much like a sponge, and with proper use of the joint we can squeeze out waste products and bring in healthy nutrients.

When Things Go Ouch in the Night (Or Day)

When your joint becomes inflamed for any reason, you experience reduced glucosamine synthesis. This is bad. The reduced synthesis is partly caused by decreased glucose, the sugar substance that is also the building block for glucosamine in the cartilage matrix. Reduced glucosamine synthesis causes you to hurt more, and the pain then leads to decreased activity and also decreased nourishment of the joint.

So What Does Glucosamine Sulfate Do, If It Works?

In theory, glucosamine sulfate that you take by mouth bypasses the traditional process of glucose to glucosamine conversion. Instead of depending on your body to transform glucose into glucosamine, you might take glucosamine sulfate supplements. In effect, you skip the "middleman." And this new glucosamine source helps build and restore the damaged cartilage meshwork.

Why Does Joint Cartilage Break Down in the First Place?

Joint cartilage breakdown can occur for a number of reasons. The usual suspects are deterioration due to normal aging, degenerative changes because of trauma, and infectious or inflammatory processes that occur for a variety of reasons. However, the end result is the same no matter what started the process: your arthritis and your arthritis pain.

As you develop arthritic inflammatory processes of the joints, not only do your joints have fewer of the building blocks to make new cartilage, but it also appears that whatever glucose/glucosamine that you do have is less efficient. It has trouble crossing the joint barrier. It's like a wounded soldier trying to make it to the front lines. As a result, your cartilage is not sufficiently replenished and it becomes more worn out and less able to repair itself.

Three things are required for a healthy joint system: (1) water; (2) a chemical substance called proteoglycans, which attracts the water like a sponge and holds it in place; and (3) collagens, which hold the proteoglycans in place.

Glucose, a sugar energy substance of the body, is converted to glucosamine, and glucosamine is ultimately converted to glycosaminoglycans, a proteoglycan for the joint cartilage.

The theory is that glucosamine, particularly glucosamine sulfate, works by bypassing the glucose conversion, particularly when body glucose is minimal or not there at all. The chondrocyte can then use glucosamine sulfate directly to make the proteoglycans, and, therefore, to preserve or repair a healthy joint cartilage.

CHONDROITIN SULFATE—WHAT IS IT?

Chondroitin sulfate is the counterpart substance to glucosamine and is recommended as an additional supplement therapy for arthritis symptom relief. It is one of many chemicals known as glycosaminoglycans or mucopolysaccarides. Some substances included in this class are shark cartilage, sea cucumber, and green-lipped mussels. All of these have, at one time or another, been touted as stand alone arthritis treatments.

Glycosaminoglycans are considered *hydrophilic,* or water loving. When combined with the proteoglycans and glucosamine, the chondroitin sulfate can act to increase the absorption of water, nutrients, and fluid substance into the joint cartilage. The effect is to make your joints a well-oiled machine. Did your arthritis ever make you feel like the Tin Man in *The Wizard of Oz,* as if you needed somebody to oil up your joints? The theory is that chondroitin is your oil can.

PROS AND CONS: A REVIEW

In *The Arthritis Solution* we looked at the pros and cons of using glucosamine and chondroitin as potential improvers of arthritis, outlining a case for and against these two natural substances. We'll cover the pros and cons here again, based on recent knowledge.

First of all, as physicians, we are sworn to the Hippocratic Oath. The first rule of medicine is Do No Harm. So it is important for us to review and analyze any therapeutic option open to us, and to make sure it is safe before we risk patient care or patient health. The review of literature of glucosamine and chondroitin sulfate studies is still difficult to interpret.

Western medical science values long-term and large-volume patient control studies. Just because these substances work for a few people doesn't mean they will work for many people. We want to see some hard data. Unfortunately, when it comes to glucosamine or chondroitin, there is very little hard data right now. The few studies that exist have used only very small numbers of people, and none of them were double-blind—both the physicians and patients knew whether the patient was receiving the chemical or not. In addition, some of the large claims made by the physicians performing the studies were not supported by statistical analysis.

For example, one study of eighty patients, forty of whom who were taking placebos (sugar pills) and the other forty who were taking glucosamine and chondroitin in combination, found that sixteen improved significantly on placebo, while twenty-two improved significantly with the glucosamine/chondroitin combination. There's not much difference between the sixteen who felt better by taking a sugar pill versus the twenty-two who felt better by taking the combination therapy.

Another question that serious people should ask is, why did some of the patients improve so dramatically in such a short period of time? Joint cartilage repair takes the body weeks or months and physically cannot occur over days. This is simply not how the body heals.

Some studies that have looked at glucosamine and chondroitin have used subjective ratings rather than X-rays, other objective ratings, or range of motion measurements. So they are using the patient's own evaluation rather than hard data.

Another area of concern is possible side effects of glucosamine and chondroitin therapy. While the studies did not cite any significant side effects, they do exist. Some side effects are rash, fluid retention, nausea, and chemical intolerance.

Lastly, there was a biochemical concern regarding these two substances: Do they really get to the root of the problem? The goal of the glucosamine and chondroitin is to get to the joint capsule through the cartilage surface and subsequently help nourish and rebuild the cartilage. But we don't know for sure if these chemicals actually arrive at the joint space.

Although it's been noted that glucosamine sulfate taken by mouth can be absorbed up to 98 percent, some estimates for absorption are as low as in the mid-range of 80+ percent absorption. However, the estimates for chondroitin sulfate absorption are quite a bit lower. Indeed, most reports cite the absorption rate from 0 to 8 percent.

The Arthritis Foundation reviewed some of these articles as well as *The Arthritis Cure,* but has elected to take a wait and see stand. The Arthritis Foundation did announce that it was unable to recommend the use of glucosamine sulfate or chondroitin sulfate as a cure for arthritis. At the same time, Dr. Doyt Conn, Senior Vice President of The Arthritis Foundation, pointed out that it is "probably not harmful, but not considered scientifically acceptable as a treatment cure."

SO WHAT DO WE THINK?

Originally, we had mixed feelings about glucosamine and chondroitin. We were bemused to learn that veterinarians have been using these two ingredients for some time with wonderful results. In addition, European physicians have been using glucosamine in particular, more than chondroitin sulfate, for arthritis pain. European results have been positive, although they are not the controlled studies desired by traditional Western medicine.

Many short-term studies have shown that the effectiveness of these two substances is equal to or greater than that of anti-inflammatory medicines such as ibuprofen.

Many short-term studies have shown that the effectiveness of these two substances is equal to or greater than that of anti-inflammatory medicines such as ibuprofen, particularly at the four-week point. But, on the plus side, the side effects from these two drugs are far less and patients tolerate these natural supplements much better than they do the traditional anti-inflammatory medicines.

Also, previously we accepted that there was very minimal, if any, risk to these natural ingredients, although those who are allergic to sulfa drugs should not take them in the sulfate form.

Although we were somewhat skeptical, we've found that often patients are the best educators. Following are just a few of the dramatic results that we have witnessed.

Tom W.

Tom W. was an active, healthy eighty-five-year-old practicing accountant. He had been putting off a left knee joint replacement for some time, having been followed by the orthopedist on a quarterly basis. In December 1996 Tom told his orthopedist, "I can't go through another busy accounting season with my knee like this. If it's not better after tax season, let's do the surgery." Tom was also seeing me (Dr. Kandel) for a back problem, and we elected to start him on the glucosamine sulfate/chondroitin sulfate regimen. I told him that this was not a proven treatment, but rather a theoretical one. Finances were not a concern to this individual, who had suffered with his left knee pain for many years.

When I saw him in May 1997, I asked Tom how the surgery went. He looked at me puzzled, asking, "Doc, what surgery?" He had walked into the exam room without his typical cane, walking straighter and looking younger than I had seen him in years. I reminded him of his plan to have his left knee "redone" with a joint replacement because of knee pain. He told me, "Doc, three months after taking those pills you recommended, my knee joint was better. Heck, even my back was better."

"Doc, three months after taking those pills you recommended, my knee joint was better. Heck, even my back was better."

Startled, I contacted the orthopedist who had done a follow-up X-ray on this patient. He told me that the cartilage was improved and that Tom no longer needed the joint replacement surgery because he had so few symptoms. A miracle cure? I don't know. But Tom thinks so.

Allison K.

Allison K was a forty-eight-year-old woman who has been a patient of Dr. Sudderth for the last four years. She suffered from severe joint pains and myofascial pain (pain in the muscles and the coverings of the muscles), and had steadily declined. Allison had seen numerous specialists, including rheumatologists, internists, and endocrinologists (hormone doctors); yet, despite all this doctoring, she continued to worsen. Allison had tried everything for her joint pain, muscle and ligament pain. No relief and the problem was getting worse.

Allison was ready and willing to try anything. She had tried chiropractic care, acupuncture, narcotic pain management, antidepressants, muscle relaxants, and sleep medications. You name it, she tried it.

In the spring of 1997, Dr. Sudderth started Allison on the glucosamine and chondroitin regimen. She had minimal improvement in her symptoms, and after two months, she was ready to "give up." However, with a little support and encouragement—as well as reminders that she hadn't experienced any negative side effects (unlike her experiences with almost all of her other prescription therapies)—Allison agreed to continue for an additional series of weeks.

After three and a half months on the regimen, Allison was markedly improved. She was getting better daily. Allison reported that she was now able to walk in her neighbor's pool for twenty minutes twice a day, whereas before to consider walking in a pool or even walking for twenty minutes a day would have been out of the question. Her overall appearance was different, her mood and energy level were much improved, and she was able to go off her prescription antidepressants.

At a six-month follow-up, it is exciting to reveal that Allison is doing better still and her last four and a half years of pain and misery are almost entirely behind her.

IF YOU WANT TO TRY THIS REGIMEN, HOW DO YOU START?

As you have seen, glucosamine and chondroitin sulfate therapy may not be a cure for everyone. But it certainly is a reasonable option in the complete picture of arthritis pain relief. So how can you get started?

First, make sure your physician is aware of the fact that you want to start taking these natural ingredients. She probably won't have an objection, and it's always nice to work with your physician as a partner in health care.

Next, where do you find glucosamine and chondroitin? These supplements are available in over-the-counter form at most natural food stores and at nutritional supplement and natural therapy centers. They are also available at many pharmacies and in some supermarkets in the supplement section.

How much is enough? The dosage that has been most studied has been glucosamine sulfate 500 mg (usually in the capsule form) to be taken three times a day. You don't have to take this with food, although if there is any nausea or bloating, taking the capsules with food may minimize this. It may also be easier to remember to take the supplement if it's taken with meals.

The chondroitin sulfate comes in 400 mg capsules. Take it three times per day, for a total of 1,200 mg per day.

A slightly higher dose is recommended for people who weigh 200 pounds or more. In individuals over age sixty-five, a slightly lower dose (1,000 mg of glucosamine per day, 800 mg of chondroitin sulfate per day) is recommended.

Be careful about where you obtain these natural supplements. Because these natural supplements aren't government controlled, their quality can vary. In one study, almost 20 percent of glucosamine/chondroitin brands contained much less than the stated amounts. In fact, some brands contained absolutely *no* glucosamine or chondroitin sulfate. We often recommend to our patients that they obtain the nutrients or supplements through a pharmacy that they are comfortable with, or through a national and respected health food store or nutritional store. Ask the store owner or pharmacist if this brand is reputable. Ask if it's a company that's been around for a few years, or a newer brand that may not be available the next time you need a refill.

Be careful about where you obtain these natural supplements. Because these natural supplements aren't government controlled, their quality can vary.

There are also combination formulations available on the market, and for the first two or three months this might be an acceptable idea. However, we routinely suggest to our patients that they obtain these chemicals separately so we can adjust the dosage if necessary.

Another word of caution: cost. Shopping around for natural supplements is worth the trouble. We have found the price in our community to range from a low of $28 per month for the glucosamine alone to nearly $200 per month, quite a shocking price difference for the same chemical. The average price is $1 to $1.50 per day for the combination, with some careful shopping and some volume buying.

A Practical Note

Exercise some patience—try not to expect immediate results. We have seen the greatest benefits with glucosamine sulfate/chondroitin sulfate at approximately three to four months. However, we do not give up on the chemicals until we have tried them for six to nine months because there may be a slow and cumulative effect. In addition, after approximately three to four months, we recommend to our patients that they use glucosamine only, because we're uncertain if there is any additional benefit of continuing with the chondroitin sulfate chemical after that period of time. There may not be a true benefit initially, yet the majority of studies have reviewed the combination of these two chemicals and we feel most comfortable (in light of the minimal cost and minimal side effects) in recommending the two chemicals together, at least initially.

A FINAL SUCCESS STORY

John R. is one of Dr. Kandel's patients. John is a wealthy entrepreneur who has the luxury of being able to afford the finest health care throughout the United States. He has his own private jet and has flown to medical appointments at the Rochester Mayo Clinic, the Cleveland Clinic, Massachusetts General Hospital, and so forth.

John has suffered from chronic back pain and bilateral hip joint pain for about eleven years. After reading one of our other books, he made an appointment to be evaluated. I examined him and ran tests and ultimately diagnosed him with spinal osteoarthritis. In addition, he also had arthritis in his hip joints.

This very frustrated patient had truly tried every medicine and therapy known to traditional science. And often he had tried them two or three times. I explained to him, as he gave me his volumes of medical records, that there might be little I could offer.

I stressed adequate diet to John, suggesting some of the recipes offered in this book. I also outlined the role of exercise in a logical and rational approach. Finally, I suggested he try the glucosamine and chondroitin sulfate regimen.

Six weeks later, he contacted me by fax to tell me that the diet was not working, he was too busy to exercise, and, of course, the supplements had been ineffective. I faxed back a note telling John that he should try these three equally important arthritis improvers for at least an additional six weeks before giving up hope. After all, he had very little to lose. I also recommended certain stretching and flexibility exercises, heat three times per day to the affected low back and hip joints, and urged him to continue the diet that I outlined.

Several months later, John was back in my office and I expected him to complain about his arthritis. To my shock, he did *both* a handstand and a cartwheel to demonstrate how much better he felt! He was beaming from ear to ear, and explained that this was the best that he had felt in almost a decade. He pointed out that he really had been ready to give up on everything. But since I had faxed him back a note urging him to keep trying, he felt that I must really believe in this regimen. So he had continued on. His personal chef made the recipes that we outlined and he did the exercises thirty to forty minutes daily with low-impact stretching and flexibility. He used the heat I'd prescribed and he continued on with the glucosamine and chondroitin.

This patient is a true convert who preaches to everyone the benefits of exercise, appropriate diet, and the use of glucosamine and chondroitin. In addition, he has mentioned throughout the country what a bright physician I am for outlining this dramatic therapeutic regimen. Don't expect this regimen to have you doing cartwheels in your doctor's office as John did! But you may feel significantly better.

This patient is a true convert who preaches to everyone the benefits of exercise, appropriate diet, and the use of glucosamine and chondroitin.

Chapter 10

THE HEALTHY LIFESTYLE

SO FAR WE'VE DISCUSSED ARTHRITIS IN GENERAL AS WELL as some basics on nutrition, and also provided you with an entire month of healthy and delicious recipes to start you on your way to improved health. These are important first steps. But in addition to knowledge about diet and learning how to eat right (and doing it!), you need to also achieve a healthy lifestyle.

We believe a healthy lifestyle means you work at three areas: eating right, maintaining a positive attitude, and exercising regularly. All three are important. If you do well in one or two of these areas but you're missing the third, you're not doing all you can to support yourself. In addition to these three standbys, you should also make sure you get a good night's sleep, and keep in mind the interaction of your mind and your body. We discuss these issues in this chapter.

A healthy lifestyle means you work at three areas: eating right, maintaining a positive attitude, and exercising regularly. All three are important.

EXERCISE: USE IT OR LOSE IT.

In his popular book *Eight Weeks to Optimum Health,* Dr. Andrew Weill strongly favors walking as the ultimate exercise. We agree that walking is a reasonable exercise—especially if the choice is between sitting on the couch and walking. Most of us can take walks with a fairly minimal degree of discomfort. Even with the discomfort of arthritis pain, many patients continue to walk.

But just walking and no other exercise is a bad idea. For example, contrary to popular belief, regular walking does *not* help your heart or your arthritis—unless the walker can increase her resting heart rate (your heart rate when you're sitting on the couch) to a certain target range (which varies from individual to individual) for twenty to forty minutes. I'm afraid some people will say, "Okay, walking's not good enough? Then I'll quit walking!" And then they'll do nothing. I think this is a valid concern.

Most of our patients are very shocked to hear us say this. Both of us have often been told by patients, "Doctor, I walk regularly, and everybody knows that's good exercise!" But when we ask for details about their walking, such as how often they walk, how far, how long, and whether or not they check their pulse for any aerobic benefit of walking, they gaze back in shock. After all, isn't walking just, well, walking?

By slowly and steadily working the knee and building the muscle, you are removing pressure from the joints. By also watching your diet and taking any needed nutrients and supplements, you will usually find that your knee joint can slowly start to repair itself.

The fact is, for exercise to provide a therapeutic benefit to increase your cardiopulmonary fitness, you really need to do either exertional activity (resistance training) or aerobic training or a combination of the two. Many personal trainers, exercise physiologists, and physical therapists recommend a combination approach. They combine aerobic activity for three days a week with strength training or resistance training for two days a week. This approach not only increases body tone but also improves the overall muscle endurance.

Here's what happens: Your body is accustomed to a certain weight load (however much you weigh). So if you walk around, you are not building up muscle tone. Instead, you are merely maintaining the current level. And if this current level is one of a debilitating arthritis, this is not a good status quo. On the other hand, progressive resistance, slowly and steadily increasing the weight, and increasing the resistance will lead to strength and endurance for the muscles themselves.

Here's an example. Let's say that your left knee is inflamed, sore, aching, and ready to give out. Let's also say that the only exercise you do is walk.

(And not too much of that.) After all, you have a sore knee. By slowly and steadily working the knee and building the muscle, particularly the muscles supporting the knee, the quadriceps, and tendons and ligaments, you are removing pressure from the joints. By also watching your diet and taking any needed nutrients and supplements, you will usually find that your knee joint can slowly start to repair itself.

It's no good to continue your same old habits, the same old routine of simply walking in a limited fashion. This won't bring the knee back to its former self, its previous health, nor will it slow the deterioration process that has already begun. You've got to use it or lose it.

It's no good to continue your same old habits, the same old routine. This won't bring the knee back to its former self, its previous health, nor will it slow the deterioration process that has already begun. You've got to use it or lose it.

Gee, Doc, Do I HAVE to Exercise?

We realize it's not enough to simply state, "Go out and exercise." We encourage our patients to find an athletic endeavor that is safe and effective for them, tailored as much as possible to their needs and lifestyles. For example, it's silly to recommend treadmill exercise if an individual despises indoor activities. Bicycling or even roller blading could be your style.

On the other hand, if you are less of a "jock," we'd be likely to start you off on a stationary bicycle, a health glider, or other form of less exertional activity. Exercise has to start somewhere, and in our earlier book, *The Arthritis Solution,* we demonstrated a number of very simple and safe stretching and range of motion flexibility exercises that can be done in the privacy of your home. No expensive fitness clothes or fancy and costly fitness equipment is required.

Do We Truly Believe in Exercise?

In January 1995 we hosted an elaborate seminar at the Ritz Carlton that was open to the community. A panel of seventeen different specialists spoke about the benefits of exercise and fitness, on both physical and emotional wellbeing. The medical specialists ranged from neurosurgeons to psychiatrists, rheumatologists, rehabilitation medicine experts and others. (And, of course, neurologists, which is our specialty.) All the physicians emphasized the tremendous value of therapeutic exercise, even a limited amount, twenty to thirty minutes three times per week.

And when you think about it, is that really such an enormous time investment? If you calculate out the hours in the week (168 hours) and subtract 1.5 hours, that leaves 166.5 hours for all other life activities, and 1.5 hours for just general fitness and exercise. This, at a minimum, would start to have a positive impact on your general health.

All the physicians emphasized the tremendous value of therapeutic exercise, even a limited amount, twenty to thirty minutes three times per week.

Over a thousand community members attended our seminar. It turned out to be a very positive learning experience not only for the general public, but also for the physicians providing the information for their specialty. For example, an oncologist (cancer doctor) discovered that exercise reduced the risk for gastrointestinal cancer and breast cancer.

A neurosurgical colleague explained that exercise speeded the healing process, reduced postoperative pain and postoperative complications, and increased the patient's subjective rating of his long-term results. Neuropsychologists and psychiatrists discussed the values of exercise, including improved memory, attention, and recall. For example, "tip of the tongue aphasia" (it's right there on the tip of my tongue) is dramatically improved with exercise. Mood and judgment are dramatically improved with exercise. Some studies indicate that physical exercise slows the cognitive decline in individuals with dementing processes such as Alzheimer's disease.

Why Don't People Love Exercising, If It's So Great?

What really is holding you back? Well, first of all, there's the pain itself. Then there are nagging doubts, "What if I exercise and hurt myself?" Finally, there is just plain old human nature. A recent study indicated that only 22 percent of people who are instructed (actually given specific instructions for exercises by their doctor, not just told to exercise) do their home exercise program. That means that a whopping 78 percent do not do their home exercises, even though it is part of a physician's complete treatment plan.

The Pain! The Pain!

With appropriate pain management, the right kind of warm-up, flexibility, heating of the affected joints, and a good exercise regimen tailored to you, pain can be minimized. Keep in mind that even though we have all heard the expression "No pain, no gain," it doesn't necessarily have to be that way.

All exercise does not have to hurt. Sure, there's going to be the discomfort and aching muscles, particularly those muscles that haven't been used for awhile. But that will quickly resolve, and can be easily treated with over-the-counter analgesics (like Tylenol) or anti-inflammatory medications. In most cases, natural therapeutic regimens, liniments, rubs, and alternative therapies are often very helpful. So using pain as a limiting excuse simply does not wash in our practice.

Fear of Hurting Yourself

Next, there's the concern of self-injury. An interesting article in the *Journal of American Geriatrics Society* (January 1996) showed that individuals who rarely exercised developed musculoskeletal injuries during exercise. Indeed, in this study there were no major injuries noted. Moderate intensity stationary exercise activity, strength training, and general fitness didn't aggravate joint symptoms in senior adults.

Another study, in the *Arthritis and Rheumatology Journal* (January 1996), showed that vigorous running did not increase musculoskeletal pain with age. Instead, researchers found a reduction in joint pain with aggressive exertional activity, such as running. In addition, active people rated their pain as being much less intense than those who did not exercise.

Active people rated their pain as being much less intense as those that did not exercise.

Exercise Is Vital to Your Health

We know some people will never be exercise enthusiasts. However, if your heart surgeon told you that your heart arteries were clogging, and you could reverse this condition with a simple exercise regimen, diet change, and lifestyle change, you might consider it. (We hope!) Especially if the alternative was an extremely risky and quite expensive bypass surgery. Wouldn't you opt for following a simpler, more conservative course? We hope most people would.

Yet many people don't understand or believe that their arthritis pain can be equally as devastating and life threatening as their heart pain or heart blood vessel disease. People who suffer from joint pains develop a downward spiral. Their pain causes them to limit their activities, which then leads to muscle weakness. This, in turn, leads to additional injury from mere everyday activities. This then leads to more pain, more limited activity, and more muscle disuse. This downward spiral is called the deconditioning spiral.

Another problem that occurs is a slowing down of your metabolism. Your joint pains increase and the pain feels more intense than it did in the past. Depression becomes a major issue. Obesity is another problem

This negative cycle can also make your blood pressure go up. If you have sugar diabetes problems, they can worsen and ultimately can lead to very serious medical consequences. So you see, you're not just exercising one joint. You're not exercising a series of joints. You're exercising your whole body, and turning your body into a fit, well-oiled machine.

THE MIND/BODY CONNECTION

You get a notice from the IRS. Before you even open the envelope, your heart starts to beat faster, you tense up in anxious anticipation, and you can feel your blood pressure rising. The same sort of physical responses to emotional stress can happen if you receive news that one of your family members is ill, or that you have an unexpected medical problem, or you go through a job change, or you're stuck in a traffic jam on the way to work. All of these negative stressors can lead to what is sometimes referred to as "toxic emotions." Toxic emotions can alter your general health and play a significant role on your overall physical and emotional well-being. Let's take a closer look.

First of all, when we are under stress, either good stress (you're excited about something nice that has happened) or bad stress, we activate our sympathetic nervous system. This is the system that gets your heart pumping, raises your blood pressure, releases stress chemicals from your adrenal gland, cuts down circulation to your stomach, and so on. Your body is getting you ready to face whatever challenge is ahead.

Unfortunately, while this branch of the nervous system is effective if you really are facing a challenging situation, a physical or exertional situation, it can also go into action over everyday occurences like those in the paragraph above. You are not in physical danger, yet your body may release the same stress chemicals as if you were truly under attack. It will also elevate your blood pressure and increase your overall body tone in a generalized readiness to act. If this process occurs many times throughout the course of the day, it's bound to take its toll on your body. When you have one of those false alarms, what you really need most is calming, soothing, reinforcing messages to your nervous system: "It's okay, just a false alarm, don't worry." Exercising can improve your ability to cope with these frequent false alarms that we all face and help you come down to normal faster.

Exercising can improve your ability to cope with daily stresses.

Psychoneuroimmunology is a branch of medicine that delves into the aspects of the mind/body connection. It seeks to explain how emotions that we experience and interpret can interact with our bodies, changing the role of the nervous system, and even affecting on a cellular level how white blood cells react to stress, infections, etc. Researchers have made some intriguing findings, including support for beliefs many of us have held for a long time. For example, we've all heard people say, "He seems run down, he's been under stress, and that's why he caught a cold." There is indeed some truth to that.

The more emotionally fit we are, the more physical fitness we attain, the better. Instead of having a downward cycle of the part of the nervous system that causes us to react, we can stimulate the parasympathetic nervous system. This is the system that helps us to relax the one that helps us to avoid harmful side effects and consequences of those toxic emotions.

Many physicians have said that just taking one day off to simply "smell the flowers" or taking pleasant strolls are valuable and important mechanisms to help you relax and reduce stress and its negative consequences.

These very simple strategies will help you emotionally unpack, to better prepare yourself for life's further emotional journeys. Many books have been written in the last few years detailing the many stress-reduction strategies we can use to slow down. If you have trouble doing this on your own, help is as close as the library.

SLEEP: NATURE'S MUSCLE CURE

We have all said at one time or another, "I know I'd feel better if I could just get a good night's sleep." We have recently learned how true this is. For example, studies on older people with sleep disorders found that exercise four times a week actually improved their sleep disorder problem. They fell asleep faster and most slept an hour more and were rested and healthy during the day. Researchers have also looked at the effects of sleep deprivation on young, healthy college students. They learned that if college students were allowed to sleep for two weeks in an uninterrupted fashion, achieving a deep restorative sleep, then they had no problems with muscle tone, muscle cramping, or muscle pain.

Studies on older people with sleep disorders found that exercise four times a week actually improved their sleep disorder problem. They fell asleep faster and most slept an hour more.

But when an additional similar matched group of college students was awakened night after night when they started to enter sleep stage 3 or 4 (deep restorative stages), after two weeks a muscle biopsy proved muscle tissue damage had occurred. So what does this tell us? It tells us that if we don't sleep well, if we don't get into the deep healing stages of sleep, then we can actually promote tissue damage.

Let's take this one step further. Imagine you are having joint pains. Night after night, month after month, you're not sleeping. We've already explained how important the supporting muscles around the joints are, to help take the burden and load off of those joints. Imagine if these muscles start to deteriorate and become inflamed. What happens to the joints? Ultimately, they have to bear more of the stress; they degenerate more quickly and you experience more discomfort and pain.

What Can You Do To Promote Positive Sleep?

First of all, establish a secure, nurturing sleep environment. That may include soothing sounds, soft music, or white noise. It may also mean a firm or extra-firm mattress on your bed and maybe a down comforter. Whatever it is, pay as much attention to your sleep environment as you would your work environment. After all, you're there in Sleepland (or should be) for almost as much time as you are awake.

And sleep should be exactly that, sleep. It shouldn't be a time to rehash the day's financial news or the day's good or bad tidings. Instead you should sleep in a place where you can restore your body to its optimum health.

But what if you can't sleep? Do you lie there, tossing and turning? Most sleep specialists explain that if you can't sleep after about fifteen or twenty minutes, then get up, get out of bed, read the paper, drink warm milk, put on soothing music, or do what ever it takes to help you get comfortable, and feel more relaxed. This is the one time when we tell you *not* to exercise! In fact, while exercise earlier in the day can promote restful sleep, vigorous exercise close to bedtime can actually interfere with your rest.

We tell our patients that not everyone needs eight solid hours of sleep every single night. Possibly if you're not sleepy when you go to bed, you may be going to bed too early. Or, you may still be finishing the day's activities in your mind, and not allowing yourself to "turn off" for the night. Here are some helpful hints you can use to prepare yourself for a good night's sleep.

Avoid Sleep Medications

Believe it or not, sleep medicines are the most common cause of insomnia. They often cause a "rebound phenomenon"—a secondary insomnia—particularly if you've depended on these medications for a long time. This is extremely difficult to treat, so avoid creating this problem before it occurs.

Keep a Sleep Diary

Often we hear from patients, "I didn't sleep at all, I haven't slept at all for the last four years!" This certainly can't be true. Our sleep cycle and our perception of our own sleeping pattern may be two very different things. If a spouse or significant other can't help you keep track of this, then a comprehensive sleep evaluation may be in order. This will help you determine the cause of the sleep problem, and the degree and severity of sleep disorder.

Sometimes, a sleep disorder can be a short-term problem, and a patient acquires a "sleep debt." This happens frequently during college finals. Students drink caffeine, take stimulants, and stay up all night to study for final exams. Afterwards, they sleep for two days, and their cycle is restored. If you can determine if you have a simple sleep debt, and can repay that debt, then the sleep disorder should be resolved.

Limit Napping

Although a thirty- to sixty-minute nap in the early afternoon is acceptable, multiple catnaps throughout the day are a bad idea. They will throw off your sleep requirement, derange the day and night cycle, and make it almost impossible for you to have a restorative, healthful sleep at bedtime. By limiting daytime napping, you can preserve the integrity of the normal day and night sleep cycle.

Don't Go to Bed Angry

This is simple to say and it is often quite difficult to practice. Realizing that this can be a problem, simply pay attention to it, and try to use some stress relaxation techniques in order to avoid this as a recurrent problem.

Avoid Stimulating Substances Prior to Bedtime

Caffeine and antihistamines (including cold medicines) can act as an irritant to the nervous system, interfering with sleep. Check with your physician to determine if any of the medications you may be taking could be having a negative effect on your sleep cycle. A review with your pharmacist would also be very helpful.

Avoid Alcohol Before Bedtime

You should avoid alcohol because of its bad effect on your joints, and nighttime alcohol is even worse. Although alcohol may help you relax initially, three to four hours after ingestion the nervous system is actually stimulated. Clearly, this can interfere with restful sleep.

Make Sure Your Environment Is Sleep Friendly

If possible, arrange your bedroom so that it is for sleeping. Move exercise equipment and computers to another room. Follow the suggestions for a calm sleeping environment we gave earlier in this chapter.

Practice Relaxation Techniques

Relaxation techniques can reduce the stress of the day, help you feel calm, and even promote drowsiness. Various breathing techniques are very helpful, not only to reduce pain, but also to provide relaxation. The suggestions below are all very effective and easy to practice at bedtime

Using calcium as a sleep aid can be as simple as drinking a glass of warm milk before bedtime.

Deep breathing is one good technique. Progressive relaxation is another that is very simple. Beginning at your feet and toes, work your way slowly up your body, progressively tensing and then relaxing each muscle. By the time you reach your trunk, chest, or upper extremities, you will likely be very drowsy, relaxed, and calm. Guided imagery or meditation are also helpful.

Natural Sleep Aids

Natural sleep aids include melatonin, vitamin B-3, calcium, and magnesium. Using calcium as a sleep aid can be as simple as drinking a glass of warm milk before bedtime, or taking your daily calcium/magnesium supplement before you go to sleep instead of in the morning. Valerian root and passionflower are two herbs with minimal negative side effects. Used cautiously and appropriately, these herbs might help with your sleep cycle.

THE LAST WORD ON LIFESTYLE

A healthy lifestyle means something different for everyone. But in general, a healthy dietary intake, routine exercise, and a healthy sleep cycle can reverse even severe symptoms and debilitating arthritis pain. This can lead in turn to a healthier and more fulfilling life. If you feel that you are better, you *are* better!

A healthy lifestyle consisting of a healthy dietary intake, routine exercise, and a healthy sleep cycle can reverse even severe symptoms and debilitating arthritis pain.

Chapter 11

COMPLEMENTARY THERAPIES FOR ARTHRITIS PAIN

SO FAR, WE'VE DISCUSSED WHAT ARTHRITIS IS, AND HOW you can take charge of your symptoms through eating the right kinds of foods, learning to deal with stress, and getting the right kind of exercise. Maybe by now you've even tried some of the wholesome, delicious, and nutritious recipes and started on your thirty-day plan for arthritis pain relief. If you're ready to take an even more active role in addressing arthritis pain and taking control of your arthritis symptom complex, this chapter is for you.

Alternative therapies may not be for everyone, but you may be surprised to find out just how mainstream some of these treatment options are.

In this chapter we'll take a look at various "alternative" or complementary treatment therapies, including healing touch, relaxation therapies, and biofeedback. We'll also review magnet therapy, and provide anecdotal information regarding some of the wonderful stories we have heard from some of our patients over the last series of months, as they have used this treatment option in alleviating much if not all of their arthritis pain. Alternative therapies may not be for everyone, but you may be surprised to find out just how mainstream some of these treatment options are.

THERAPEUTIC MASSAGE

Massage therapy has been used through the ages, in many forms, to treat both acute and chronic pain. Massage can be quite effective in reducing muscle spasm and increasing circulation to affected areas, and in increasing the elimination of waste products through the lymphatic system.

MASSAGE TRIGGERS NATURAL PAIN KILLERS

Your skin surface has numerous sensory receptors. Triggering these receptors with massage therapy can initiate the healing process. This is particularly true of those areas of your body that have been blocked from the normal body healing process because of chronic tension, pain, or spasm.

Massage can also be extremely helpful in reducing the need for pain medication. The exact mechanism for why and how this happens is not entirely known. However, the theory is that massage can trigger the release of the body's own natural morphine-like substances, endorphins, which act as natural painkillers.

Massage can be extremely helpful in reducing the need for pain medication.

Therapeutic massage has been useful in obstetrics and gynecology, particularly during childbirth, and it is now finding its way even into the most traditional and mainstream of hospital facilities. Massage therapy can be extremely helpful when combined with other treatment techniques.

NEUROMUSCULAR MASSAGE

There are many different types of massage, and describing each and every type of massage therapy is beyond the scope of this text. The most common technique is Swedish massage, a form of massage therapy that promotes relaxation. But the most common type of massage used in the treatment of arthritis pain is *neuromuscular massage.*

In neuromuscular massage, the muscles and their coverings (the fascia) are released through stretching, relaxation techniques, and by deeply stimulating the muscles. Both Swedish and neuromuscular massage have significant therapeutic benefits. But when it comes to arthritis pain relief, neuromuscular massage—while perhaps not as gentle as Swedish—is much more effective. For more information on neuromuscular massage, contact a licensed massage therapist near you.

Some Pain Before the Gain

Massage therapy can sometimes produce some muscle pain and soreness, particularly after the first one or two sessions. One factor is the release of accumulated waste in the muscle tissue. These waste materials are actually being manually released during the course of massage therapy.

Another factor is that when the muscles are tight, in spasm, and inflamed, direct contact by the massage therapist can be interpreted as painful. We often describe this soreness as similar to the type of muscle ache or pain that comes when you start a new exercise or workout program, particularly if you have been a "couch potato" for a long time. But don't worry! The discomfort that may come with your new massage therapy should diminish and resolve entirely after the first few treatments.

Before and After Massage Suggestions

Warm your muscles before your massage appointment. This will help them be more elastic and pliable, allowing the therapist to get a deeper massage with less tissue inflammation.

After your massage, drink as much water as possible to help eliminate the released toxins from your system and help ease post-massage aching. In addition, applying cold therapy or ice therapy to the treated area for fifteen or twenty minutes after the massage will often be very effective. This helps reduce soreness as well as any potential post-muscle release spasm.

HYPNOSIS

Hypnosis therapy has been badly misrepresented by Hollywood movies. Many people think that if you are hypnotized, then you are under someone's "power" and can be induced to do just about anything, including acts you would normally never do. But in reality, hypnotherapy is quite different. A physician or therapist cannot "gain control of your mind." Instead, hypnotherapy can be a wonderful technique to allow you to take control of your own mind!

Hypnosis is *always* "self-hypnosis." In other words, it is the patient who achieves the hypnotic state of mind, while the therapist acts only as a guide. Clearly, you cannot be hypnotized against your will.

How does it work? You are trained to create a state of highly focused attention and then to ultimately reach a point of complete relaxation. By accomplishing this goal, you can achieve a significant reduction in pain, perhaps even total elimination of pain.

Learning Self-Hypnosis Before Acute Pain Strikes

It can be difficult to hypnotize yourself when you are in the throes of an acute attack of pain. For this very reason, we don't wait until the last minute to teach our patients how to do self-directed hypnosis therapy. Rather, we try to teach them how to modify their own behavior, how to appreciate the onset of pain, and how to perform hypnotherapy on themselves *before* an acute attack. Self-hypnosis can help you stop an acute attack so it does not become the major event (or the only event) in your day.

More on Self-Hypnosis

Hypnosis is a form of focused attention. By focusing on certain aspects of the environment, such as a cool breeze, a breathing pattern, or a peaceful sound, you can learn to shift the focus away from your severe arthritis pain.

Self-hypnosis can help you stop an acute attack so it does not become the major event in your day.

This is not only a subjective determination. In our clinic we have used temperature probes to discover that patients who have learned to use hypnosis effectively can actually "cool off" an inflamed joint, particularly when there is acute pain. If fact, some can alter the body temperature of their affected joints by as much as three to seven degrees! They can also learn to use hypnotherapy to warm up areas of the body, to increase circulation, and to help expedite the removal of waste products.

Simply put, they are using their mind to control their body's temperature, almost using their mind as a form of physical therapy to do heat and ice therapy. This is remarkable, considering there is no heat or ice being used to alter the temperature of the limbs.

We have used temperature probes to discover that patients who have learned to use hypnosis effectively can actually "cool off" an inflamed joint, particularly when there is acute pain.

Hypnosis therapy can take time to master, so don't expect to be an expert in an hour or a day. However, with practice, it becomes easier and easier. Eventually, you should be able to enter into a mild trance state in a very short period of time. Often, patients can enter a state of calm, and then arouse themselves after two to three minutes, with a significant reduction in their rating of pain following these brief sessions.

BREATHING THERAPIES

Every human knows how to breathe, right? Wrong! While we do breathe in and out every minute of every day, very few people actually take the time or pay the appropriate attention to their breathing technique. For example, are you breathing in and out in a slow deliberate pattern? Are you taking deep breaths? And when you're hurting, do you pay any attention whatsoever to your breathing pattern?

Rapid Breathing Can Escalate Pain

It is natural to withdraw into yourself when you are having pain. Most of us tend to contract our muscles and not expand our lungs. This results in small, shallow breaths that in turn lead to rapid breathing. This rapid breathing cycle can actually start a hyperventilation syndrome: Small shallow breaths don't provide enough oxygen to the brain, so the brain triggers more rapid breathing to make up for this. Rapid, shallow breathing can actually escalate the cycle of pain, particularly when this rapid breathing is combined with an increased heart rate and escalating rates of adrenaline (the fight or flight chemicals in our body). But you can take control of this pattern and stop it in its tracks.

How? With simple deep breathing techniques. When you breathe slowly and deeply, your body can actually draw in enough oxygen with each breath to allow the brain to relax and the breathing pattern to normalize. This then shifts the focus away from the stress reaction and back into the calming, or relaxation, mode.

Rapid, shallow breathing can actually escalate the cycle of pain, but you can take control of this pattern and stop it in its tracks.

Your nervous system is a very complex system of feedback and reaction mechanisms. When one act occurs, it triggers other changes in your body, and if these are acts that stimulate the body (such as rapid breathing, causing increased heart rate and so forth), this is not good for the person with arthritis and can increase your pain. But with focused concentration, attention to deep breathing, and slow and deliberate breaths, you can activate a positive feedback loop. This positive feedback loop can trigger your natural relaxation chemicals and cause them to be released into the bloodstream. These biochemicals ultimately allow the body to relax, and the end result is decreased pain.

As with many good things, the more that good deep breathing techniques are practiced, the more they become a natural and unconscious response. Even when brief attacks of arthritis pain flare up, the breathing technique, which is ingrained as a response pattern of slow deep breathing and focused attention, will allow the body to naturally shift away from acknowledging and reacting to the severe pain.

What Is Correct Breathing?

Diaphragmatic breathing, commonly referred to as a deep breathing, is not hard to learn. Begin your breathing exercises in a calm, quiet, and relaxed environment. Dr. Kandel often reminds his patients to try deep breathing when the pain is mild, and not wait until the pain is severe.

Close your eyes and inhale deeply and slowly. Mentally count a slow and steady one, two, three, four as you continue to inhale. Then hold your breath lightly for a moment and count four, three, two, one, as you slowly exhale. Then repeat the cycle.

During the deep breathing, be aware of where the air is going. Are you expanding your abdominal muscles, filling your stomach with air? You are aiming for diaphragmatic breathing, so focus on filling your lungs and expanding your ribcage with each inhalation.

Even when brief attacks of arthritis pain flare up, the breathing technique will allow the body to naturally shift away from acknowledging and reacting to the severe pain.

If you're slightly too anxious to practice this type of breathing therapy on a regular basis, you may need to reinforce or even learn this technique with other tools, such as biofeedback, discussed below. Remember, everyone functions at a slightly different metabolic rate, and everyone's breathing pattern, heart rate pattern, and learning pattern are different.

However you get there, try to incorporate deep breathing into your daily routine. It is important to practice good deep diaphragmatic breathing not just occasionally, or even once a day. Rather, you should practice for seconds or minutes every hour or every few hours. It's worth it! Three minutes every two hours is really not too much to ask to provide for deep relaxation therapy, improved circulation, reduced waste products, and increased mental alertness. In addition, this is a great way to take a break from their day from your environment, your boss, your kids, and other daily stresses. Once you master this technique, you'll find that it is quite simple to perform.

RELAXATION THERAPY

It's worth it! Three minutes every two hours is really not too much to ask to provide for deep relaxation therapy, improved circulation, reduced waste products, and increased mental alertness.

How do you relax? For everyone, it's something different. For some people, it's knitting or crocheting. For others, it's watching sports. For others, it's a leisurely stroll or a walk by the beach. While these are all reasonable relaxation techniques, there's a very specific type of therapy called "progressive relaxation" that can be very helpful in reducing arthritis pain.

Progressive relaxation is easy to learn and easy to perform, even for a beginner. Progressive relaxation is actually an extension of deep breathing, but it involves all of the muscles. The idea of this treatment is to progressively contract then relax each individual muscle and then each muscle group in a methodical fashion, from toes to scalp. Here's how to do it:

You are going to contract each muscle for ten to thirty seconds, and then slowly release the contraction. As you work, focus only on the muscle you are contracting. Begin with the toes, move to the feet, to the calves, to the thighs, to the buttocks. Then move upward, to the abdomen, the diaphragm, the ribcage, the shoulders. Now do your fingers, hands, and up your arms. End with the neck, the face, and the scalp. The first time you do it, you will be amazed at how much more relaxed you feel right away.

This is not an instant therapy; it can take several minutes to achieve a calm state or a state of significant relaxation. However, it can be very effective, and combined with deep breathing, it can bring a great deal of pain relief. Over time, progressive relaxation becomes easier and easier to perform. You will discover shortcuts that allow for pain relief without requiring as much time. Since this therapy requires no special tools or equipment, you can practice it anytime and any place.

GUIDED IMAGERY

Guided imagery is a combination of hypnotherapy, deep breathing, and muscle relaxation. You imagine a calm, relaxing scene, such as drifting on the waves of the ocean, floating on the breeze, or picturing yourself in a calm, quiet, safe environment. This triggers the brain to release certain "relaxation chemicals" and to prevent the release of "stress chemicals." Ultimately, there is a release of pain-blocking chemicals from the brain. All of this acts to provide a great deal of pain relief and muscle relaxation.

Guided imagery works best when you use an image that resonates with you personally. For example, Paul was a middle-aged farmer. He was not formally educated, but was always very cooperative with any therapeutic intervention that was offered for his arthritis pain. He had tried and failed with many traditional therapies, and could not tolerate some of the anti-inflammatory or pain medicines. The medications always led to stomach upset, to sedation, or to other side effects that prevented him from doing his normal work.

Paul was referred to us by his family physician. He had exhausted the traditional treatment regimen and felt that Paul might benefit from a pain management specialist. Paul was very interested in trying pain management and treatment without pain pills.

After the initial evaluation, it was clear that Paul had a passion for sports, particularly baseball. He couldn't continue to play, not only because of his time commitments, but also even more importantly because of his joint pain. Nevertheless, he liked being a spectator and loved to watch the sport. He knew everything there was about baseball. He could name all of the players on most of the teams, could recite each individual player's statistics, and could provide use with more information about baseball than we ever really needed to know!

We began Paul's therapy session by asking him to close his eyes and picture a baseball diamond. Then I asked Paul to imagine a game in his mind, between two of his favorite teams. I asked Paul to take slow deep breaths, visualizing the stance of each and every player. I asked him to describe the weather, whether there was a breeze, and to provide any and all information and details regarding the baseball game.

At first, Paul was self-conscious. But after a few minutes, he forgot all about being in the examining room, forgot all about his arthritis pain, and indeed became quite animated. If I hadn't interrupted him, I believe I would gotten full innings from Paul. After the session, Paul felt very relaxed. On a scale of 1 to 10, his subjective rating of his pain dropped from 9 to 3. Not only that, the difference was obvious to people who observed him. The way he walked and his overall range of motion seemed to improve.

Most important, Paul realized that he was able to do this without pain pills, without shots, without needles, and without mechanical appliances. This was something he could do at work without having to take time away from his busy schedule.

Recently, Paul told me that he has learned to visualize shorter innings. This seems to be almost as effective as visualizing an entire game, and he has learned how to fine tune his imagery concentration.

Not everybody responds as well as Paul did. Guided imagery, very much like deep breathing, hypnosis, and other relaxation therapies, requires a bit of practice. As with the other treatments, it is best to learn this during a relatively pain-free interval, to allow the body to relax to its fullest, in preparation for a future painful event.

MEDITATION

Meditation is another type of relaxation therapy along the lines of deep breathing, guided imagery, and hypnosis. When you bring your awareness to a tone, a sound, a phrase, your focus naturally and easily moves away from your joint pain.

Meditation is helpful not only in alleviating pain, but also in increasing relaxation, reducing stress, increasing energy, and producing an overall sense of calm. Meditation can help you slow your heart rate, change your breathing pattern, change your body temperature, and even slow down your metabolism. Some studies have shown that meditation therapy actually alters brain-wave patterns; and chemical studies have found that this technique is often associated with an increase in the body's excretion of relaxation chemicals.

A host of recent research studies have found that meditation can produce a number of positive benefits, including improved energy, improved vigor, less fatigue, increased stamina, and decreased self-rating of pain. Also, some studies have found that people who meditate have a more natural and healthy sleep cycle, and a reduction in harmful habits such as alcohol, caffeine, and tobacco use. Most important, studies have clearly shown that meditation is very effective in reducing your pain, particularly your arthritis pain.

Meditation therapy actually alters brain-wave patterns; and is associated with an increase in the body's excretion of relaxation chemicals.

You can choose from a variety of meditation techniques. Most meditators advise learning to meditate in a group rather than on your own. You'll want the support and encouragement of others when you begin. Meditation requires anywhere from five to thirty minutes, and can be shortened as you master the technique.

YOGA

The word *yoga* might make you think of someone wearing a towel and contorting his body into an impossible looking and weird position. But you do not have to learn how to twist yourself into a pretzel to perform yoga. In fact, yoga is a unique and learnable activity that is therapeutic in its own right and has been reported as being helpful for many types of illnesses and disorders. Yoga involves minimal risk, particularly if done under careful supervision.

There are a number of varieties of yoga, but the basic concept is to perform stretching and flexibility activities in a calm and deliberate setting. This allows the body to strengthen the major muscles, the supporting muscles of the joints, increase the overall stability of the body, and relax at the same time. Stretching exercises work much like squeezing and releasing a sponge: They bring nutrients into the joint and remove waste products. In the very simplest of terms, yoga therapy helps to lubricate the joints and allows them to function in a more effective and efficient fashion.

Performing yoga on a routine basis can lead to increased range of motion and decreased pain, and to increased strength and stamina of the supporting muscles. When the supporting muscles have increased strength and function, there is less stress on the joints and ultimately less degeneration of the joints themselves. Yoga is combined with breathing techniques, and therefore this also leads to improved pain relief, increased relaxation, and decreased pain.

Performing yoga on a routine basis can lead to increased range of motion and decreased pain, and to increased strength and stamina of the supporting muscles.

One note of caution: Start slowly! When our patients start a yoga program, particularly those with severe joint pains, their range of motion is structurally limited. It is going to take weeks or months to improve the range of motion and flexibility, and often our patients overestimate their abilities. Yoga feels good at the time it is being done, so it is quite easy to overdo it. Be satisfied with small gains rather than frustrated over what you can't do. Yoga, just like any other form of true exercise, takes time, instruction, and patience to master. However, the benefits that can be obtained certainly warrant the investment of training, as another wonderful non-narcotic, non-medication therapeutic intervention.

CRYOTHERAPY: ICE IT

One of the first things that we learn when we are young is that if we sprain our ankle, our knee, or another joint, we put ice on it. This is also appropriate therapy for acute exacerbations of joint pain for patients who suffer from arthritis. *Cryotherapy* simply means the application of cold to painful and or swollen/inflamed areas. When you apply an ice pack, you are using cryotherapy.

When do you use heat, and when do you use ice? It all depends on what stage an injury is in. A rule of thumb is that for an acute inflammatory process, acute pain or sprain or muscle spasm, ice is effective over the first twelve to twenty-four hours. Afterwards, applying heat can start the healing cycle.

Whenever there is inflammation, swelling, and release of pain chemicals, applying cryotherapy can cause the blood vessels to constrict and thereby reduce the swelling and the flow of inflammatory chemicals (cytokines) to the inflamed area. Once the swelling starts to go down, muscle spasm can also be reduced. Applying cold also activates the large nerve fibers, blocking the transmission of pain messages from the small nerve fibers. This is one of the original theories of pain management, and the techniques of "blocking pain" are still used today by most pain specialists.

In addition to simply applying cold to the effective area, cold combined with massage (ice massage) can often increase function and reduce pain. One such technique is called "spray and stretch": First, a cooling spray, almost an anesthetic spray, is used on the muscles, allowing the muscles to cool and reducing spasm. Then a physician or a physical therapist stretches the muscles. This allows the muscles to relax out of the spasm. As the cooling spray wears off, the muscles start to warm, felt as a heating sensation of the joint or muscle. This is often quite effective immobilizing inflamed joints such as the hip, knee or ankle, or even the shoulder.

Like all therapies, cryotherapy needs to be used in moderation and should be performed under supervision. A rule of thumb is to leave the ice therapy or cold therapy in place no longer than fifteen to twenty minutes. After that period of time, the blood vessels involuntarily open, and this can lead to a burning of the muscles and the skin. We have our patients use ice therapy on for twenty minutes, off for one to two hours, and then repeating this cycle. This seems to be fairly effective in treating acute pain.

HEAT THERAPY

Heat therapy, of course, is exactly the opposite of cryotherapy. To see how popular heat therapy is today, you need go no further than your local pharmacy and look at the many different brands of heating creams, rubs, and lotions on the shelves.

Heat therapy is popular because it opens the blood vessels, speeds the healing process, and carries away metabolic waste products. Heat also seems to provide nourishment through the improved circulation to the inflamed muscles, which speeds tissue healing. Also, as any athlete can attest, heat applied for twenty to thirty minutes to a muscle region seems to make the muscles more elastic. With this, there is less risk of muscle damage with joint usage.

Heat can be applied moist or dry. The moist heat seems to be more effective for the major joints, although moist heat, dry heat, and heating creams all seem to be fairly effective. Moist heat can be applied through special heating pads, hot showers, and whirlpool baths.

Cold treatment seems to be helpful for the acute inflammatory process, while heat seems to be more effective for medium- and long-term management and to promote healing. Apply heat for thirty to forty minutes, then off for an hour, then repeat the cycle. Heating creams or rubs can be used four to six times a day.

If you are looking for a heating cream, ask the pharmacist for the house brand. It is usually much less expensive than the other creams, and probably doesn't have the "doctor's office" smell that some of the traditional medications have. You want pain relief, but you may not want everyone to smell you when you walk in the room. Odorless creams are just as effective as strong smelling ones.

MAGNETIC THERAPY

Everything old seems new again. This applies to attitudes, fashions, diets, and just about everything that we take part in. Magnets are no exception. Cleopatra wore magnetic bracelets, anklets, or amulets thousands of years ago. She is only one of many who believed in the power of magnetic therapy to reduce pain and speed the healing process. Today, some people are convinced that they have "discovered" the therapeutic benefit of magnet treatment.

Magnetic therapy uses the concept of biologically active and effective magnets. This is not the simple north south–directed magnet polarity; it is a different type of magnetic field. According to the concept of biologically active magnets, negative polarity predominates and actually seems to improve healing. This is true not only on an individual cell, but also on the total body basis.

Most of us have had a positive "magnetic experience." For example, the last time you sat by a quiet stream or brook, or in front of the ocean's pounding surf, you most likely felt calm, relaxed, and refreshed as your day's cares floated away. Why? Is it just the water, or is there something else? One theory holds that there are increased positive/negative ions surrounding these bubbling brooks and flowing streams, and in some way these enhance our own body energy fields: providing positive energy, restoring our sense of wellness, and re-balancing our body.

Similarly, when we sit in an oxygen-enriched environment, such as a forest, we also seem to feel refreshed. Some theorize that the increased oxygen content of the air along with the increase in positive magnetic ions mean a greater supply of oxygen-rich blood cells coursing through our body. This allows more nutrition, more oxygen, and more energy to each individual cell, and to the muscles and joints in general. Apparently, this can lead to decreased pain and increased mobility.

SCIENTIFIC STUDIES

Is there any scientific evidence that magnetic therapy can actually work? I'm glad you asked that question! At the Johns Hopkins Treatment Pain Center, researchers performed a controlled study on magnetic therapy.

In this study, some patients with chronic pain were treated to placebo therapy (like a sugar pill, there is no true benefit to a placebo), while other individuals were provided magnetic therapy. Initially, both groups of patients improved. The individuals using placebo therapy improved slightly, but this effect rapidly tapered off. Those who received the magnets, however, showed dramatic improvement. They had increased function, increased range of motion, decreased pain, and their subjective rating of their pain stayed reduced. The fact that there were no negative side effects to magnetic therapy makes this a very reasonable choice for individuals who have either failed traditional therapy, or who have rejected traditional therapy.

Researchers at the Johns Hopkins Treatment Pain Center performed a controlled study on magnetic therapy. Patients who received the magnets showed dramatic improvement.

(It should be pointed out, however, that not all types of magnetic treatment may be free of side effects. For example, right now there is controversy as to whether or not high pulsating magnetic pollution, such as seen around high power transmission lines, can produce harmful side effects. While this has not been proven, a number of anecdotal studies and case reports have been cited, with problems including such things as memory loss, headaches, changes in heart rhythm, and altered blood chemistry.)

Uses of Magnetic Therapy

How have physicians used magnetic therapy? One orthopedic surgeon has used magnetic technology in combination with traditional surgical intervention. The rates of healing for bone fracture (particularly those that are not well connected) have been greater than 80 percent, while traditional rates are much lower without magnetic therapy.

There is not a single physician practicing today who does not value the benefits of magnetic science, although he or she may discount magnetic therapy for arthritis pain. Magnetic resonance imaging scanners (MRIs) are provide diagnostic information daily on a wide variety of illnesses. MRIs are very important for assessing joints and cartilage, and are particularly effective for assessing the nervous system, such as the brain and the spinal cord. However, we find it interesting that when the topic comes up of adjusting magnetic polarity for healing purposes for our bodies, many doctors are extremely skeptical.

As this is "a new field," actually a rediscovered field of medical science, at this time anecdotal stories abound. Some stories describe athletes who have increased their stamina, exercise endurance, and even weight lifting or weight training ability through the use of magnets. A recent article in *American Pain Journal* described how magnet therapy may be helpful for neuropathy, inflammation of the nerve twigs, most often found in the lower extremities.

Anecdotal Stories

We are traditional physicians, and understand that these anecdotal stories are not the same as scientific research. But we certainly do not deny the claim that many people have improved, and often dramatically, with the assistance of magnetic therapy.

Stan, a patient of Dr. Kandel, was bed-ridden for five days because of acute joint pain in the low back and sacroiliac region. He was unable to sit or stand, and had to stay in bed. Upon hearing this, a neighbor provided him with magnetic pads: a bed pad, a low back magnetic pad, and two magnetic rollers to be used over the low back region.

Stan contacted our office, stating he did not need an emergent follow-up visit, as he was doing "great, just great." Apparently, by sleeping on the magnetic mattress, using the magnetic pads and the rollers, he had improved his symptom complex. How this works is uncertain, at least to us, despite extensive review of the literature. There are many theories, but clearly the fact remains, that our patients have been helped by the use of magnetic therapy.

One version of magnetic therapy is to alternate the pressure points of the body using the magnets. In this way, possibly, we are dealing with magnetic acupressure or a variant of magnetic acupuncture. A number of human and animal studies show that this procedure seems to provide a great deal of pain relief, particularly in various animal models, for the muscles and ligaments as well as for the joints.

Articles in clinical orthopedic journals describe patients with failed low back fusions who experience chronic pain. A number of these individuals have tried magnet therapy, and actually have experienced increased fusion benefits and reduced pain. Further studies are warranted to follow up on this very exciting field of magnetic therapy.

Neurologists also treat a number of individuals with facial pain. Many of these have tried various types of treatment, including pain medicines, antidepressant medicines, and electric stimulation. A number of our patients treated with magnetic therapy combined with electric stimulation therapy seemed to have improved dramatically, as compared to those who have been treated only with medications.

Magnets have been studied for their effects on various areas of the body, including neck and shoulder stiffness, low back pain, muscle pain, and for our purposes, joint and arthritic conditions. Individual results have varied, based on the location where the magnets have been applied, the length of time that they were used, and the patient's initial attitude (those with positive attitudes seemed to do better than those who were doubtful). The patients' subjective rating of pain reduction ranged from 56 percent to 98 percent improvement with the use of magnetic therapy. The magnetic mattress was reported to be particularly effective, and no negative side effects were found.

Types of Magnets

Magnets come in all strengths and are marketed by many different companies. We are not distributors, and we have no financial interest in any of these products, but we have had our greatest success with Nikken magnetic pads. The pads can come as small strips, pads, or larger strips to be placed on the low back region.

Magnetic balls can be used for hand therapy, very much like traditional hand therapy for arthritis joint pain. However, with the additional healing power of the magnets, people seem to have increased function, increased sense of warmth, and more rapid reduction of their pain. Their pain relief also seems to last for longer periods of times, even after brief sessions of therapy.

We were quite impressed by one study that tested the effectiveness of magnetic belts. This study used subjects suffering from low back pain and was a double-blind study (the patients and the doctors were both unaware of who was receiving the treatment or the placebo). The patients who had either no magnets or weak magnets failed to show any significant benefit. Those however who did receive the high field magnetic belt reported dramatic improvement in their low back pain.

Is it expensive? As health care expenses go, magnetic therapy can run from the gamut from relatively inexpensive to relatively expensive. One of our favorite forms of magnetic treatment are "mag steps," a relatively low-cost item. These are large, oversized shoe inserts, with bumps on one side and indentations on the other.

When they are used, they need to be trimmed to your foot's natural dimension. Some people prefer wearing these with the bumps up, others with the bumps down. There is neither a right nor wrong way to wear these inserts. Individuals who use them seem to report less leg cramping, more stability of gait and balance, less frequent falls, less unsteadiness. They also state that they have increased stamina and are able to perform activities for longer periods of time.

At the other end of the cost spectrum, there are magnetic bed pads, ranging between $450 and $600. These seem to help when there are multiple areas that need to be addressed, not just individual joints. Another very popular item with our patients are "mag boys," small hand-held magnetic balls that can be very effective for hand pain or joint pain in the fingers. A holder offered by some vendors can turn these two magnetic balls into a type of rolling massager, to be used over other parts of the body.

The Bottom Line

When all is said and done, we must admit we still don't fully understand the mechanism of magnetic therapy, how it works, or even why it works. We simply see the results.

When we discuss this with our traditional colleagues, many belittle magnetic therapy as nothing more than sham or placebo treatment. However, we point out that the proof is in the results, and our patients do well. We feel that we are treating a person with an illness rather than an illness in a person.

Because this is one more type of therapy that enlists the patient's cooperation, it allows the patients to become partners in their health care, and we think this is very important. Your doctor can't always be there when you suffer a pain spasm. In addition, having the patient as an ally, rather than a passive observer in their health care is something of great value, whether it is an arthritis pain or any other medical illness.

We have often found one additional and very important benefit of magnetic therapy. If the patients are willing to go through the routine and even the bother of putting on magnetic pads, or placing a magnetic belt in place, they often are reminded to take the time to use proper body mechanics, to be aware of their joint pain, and actually to follow through on their additional physician instructions, such as stretching and flexibility. Most important, it helps them see that they are in control of their pain syndrome. This itself might be worth the cost of a magnetic pad.

BIOFEEDBACK

Biofeedback is often extremely helpful for our patients with moderate to severe arthritis complaints. It teaches patients to observe how their body reacts to various positive and negative thoughts, and enables them to train their body to react in a way that decreases pain.

By observing the readings on special monitors that provide visual feedback on your body temperature, pulse rate, and breathing patterns, you can actually learn to change and reduce your pulse rate, calm your breathing pattern, and, best of all, increase your control over the pain from arthritis. And all without using medication.

Sometimes it can be quite difficult to master biofeedback. It requires training, dedication, and the appropriate equipment.

A Definition

Biofeedback is a technique that uses mechanical feedback to teach people how they can use their mind to alter body processes. It provides startling evidence of the mind-body connection in practice, especially for skeptics.

When you are very distraught, your pulse rate speeds up, as does your breathing. When you are calm, your pulse is slower and so is your respiration. These are natural processes that you don't really think about. In fact, you probably thought you had no control over your mind and certainly over your own natural body processes such as breathing. But maybe people do gain this very control and you may be one of them!

Biofeedback is a technique that uses mechanical feedback to teach people how they can use their mind to alter body processes. It provides startling evidence of the mind-body connection in practice, especially for skeptics.

With biofeedback, you do learn to gain control of some of these behaviors that you probably always regarded as *not* within your control. How? While hooked up to the equipment, patients are taught to think about various activities, settings, and conditions.

Controls, such as tones or beeps, measurement of skin response (the galvanic skin response measurement actually measures electrical conductivity of the skin), and other indicators are all displayed on a monitor for the patient to receive exactly the kind of feedback they need to help them modify their thoughts, energy, and focus of attention.

First, the Happy Thoughts

At first, positive environments and activities are used to produce a calming effect. This calming effect then is measured by such equipment as an EKG monitor, pulse rate monitor, or temperature probe. The patient is told to think about a pleasant event such as a nice restful day at a lake or another happy and calm day in her life. The image is one of serenity, peace, and happiness. As you envision this scene, you can actually see your heart slow down, your pulse decrease, and your breathing pattern or respiratory rate slow down. You've actually gained control over your body!

Then the Stressful Thoughts

Once you've learned how to calm yourself and your various body processes, you "graduate" to a higher level of biofeedback. (How many sessions required to achieve the calming ability varies from person to person but usually takes at least a few sessions.)

In the next stage of biofeedback, you are told to think of heart-pounding and anxiety-producing events so that you will speed up your pulse and heart rate. The technician isn't trying to torture you, but instead wants to help you first feel then stress and then master it. You use the training you've gained through biofeedback to calm your pulse, breathing, and so forth.

Biofeedback and Pain Control

The role of biofeedback in pain control is to train patients with acute and chronic pain to shift their mind's focus away from their pain and onto more pleasurable situations. This triggers the relaxation phase. As a result, more pain-controlling chemicals can be released and less stress causing chemicals are released.

Your muscles don't tighten up as much and a cascade of positive events occur, ultimately making you feel better. In addition, as mentioned with other forms of relaxation therapy, this exercise leads to a shift of focus away from the inflamed or arthritic joint.

The key benefits of biofeedback: improved oxygen in the bloodstream, improved blood circulation, decreased waste products in the body, and decreased stress. These are all interpreted by your body as decreased pain.

Are You a "Type A" Person?

Biofeedback is often very helpful for individuals who are "Type A"—"show me" or "prove it" people who require external validation of what is going on. This is an ideal technique for someone who needs to have a formal objective measurement of their success. The patient can literally see their heart rate slowing down, can see their temperature changing right in front of their eyes, and this then is reinforcing. With the continued reinforcement, and success, patients want to continue this treatment, and they actually end up obtaining excellent therapeutic benefits.

Benefits of Biofeedback

When you succeed with biofeedback, as many people have, there are many, many benefits. Here are the key benefits: improved oxygen in the bloodstream, improved blood circulation, decreased waste products in the body, and decreased stress. These are all interpreted by your body as decreased pain.

EEG Biofeedback

We have recently received additional specialty training in a new form of biofeedback, called EEG biofeedback. In this type of biofeedback, the patient is actually hooked up to a brain-wave monitor, an electroencephalogram (EEG). Neurologists have used this EEG tool for some time, measuring brain activity in patients with seizures, with migraine, etc.

Using the EEG as a biofeedback device, however, enables patients to actually see their own brain-wave activity, and to learn to change their actual brain-wave patterns. There are certain types of patterns that are more effective, particularly in obtaining a state of calm.

By obtaining a deeper more harmonious rhythm, patients can reach this level of calm. What is exciting is that once learned, you can later reproduce this effect, even though you're not hooked up to the brain-wave machine.

How? Simply by mentally recreating the relaxing environment or focus that allowed you to create those nice brain-wave patterns when you were hooked up to the machine. In other words, patients are taught what images, what pictures, what relaxation measures work for them while they are on a monitor or external device, and ultimately they transfer this learning to when they are not attached to equipment. The end result is the same.

Biofeedback as a Medical Therapy

Biofeedback is a type of therapeutic intervention that takes training and dedication, but with a patient who is motivated and cooperative, the success can be phenomenal. The National Headache Foundation recently has outlined biofeedback as an ideal choice for headache management, and we have found biofeedback to work exceptionally well for our patients with neck and back pain and joint pain associated with arthritis.

Biofeedback is one more technique that empowers patients to become active participants in their health care, while they do not require ongoing medication management, nor are they having any negative side effects of narcotic or anti-inflammatory medicines in their system.

In this chapter we have discussed various therapies that are helpful for a complete approach to arthritis care. These therapies are not meant to be used exclusively; rather, a combination of these approaches may be of greatest benefit. Each individual will have to pick and choose different therapies that work best for him or her.

As you can see, this book is dedicated to a total lifestyle approach to managing and treating arthritis pain. We hope that you will review and follow our menu plan, approach exercise with a positive attitude, and utilize the various therapeutic techniques that are complementary in treating and beating arthritis pain.

This book is a first step on the road to recovery, healing, and wellness.

TO YOUR HEALTH!

Index

C

D

H

I

J

K

L

INTERNATIONAL CONVERSION CHART

These are not exact equivalents: they've been slightly rounded to make measuring easier.

Liquid Measurements

American	*Imperial*	*Metric*	*Australian*
2 tablespoons (1 oz.)	1 fl. oz.	30 ml	1 tablespoon
1/4 cup (2 oz.)	2 fl. oz.	60 ml	2 tablespoons
1/3 cup (3 oz.)	3 fl. oz.	80 ml	1/4 cup
1/2 cup (4 oz.)	4 fl. oz.	125 ml	1/3 cup
2/3 cup (5 oz.)	5 fl. oz.	165 ml	1/2 cup
3/4 cup (6 oz.)	6 fl. oz.	185 ml	2/3 cup
1 cup (8 oz.)	8 fl. oz.	250 ml	3/4 cup

Spoon Measurements

American	*Metric*
1/4 teaspoon	1 ml
1/2 teaspoon	2 ml
1 teaspoon	5 ml
1 tablepoon	15 ml

Oven Temperatures

Fahrenheit	*Centigrade*	*Gas*
250	120	1/2
300	150	2
325	160	3
350	180	4
375	190	5
400	200	6
450	230	8

Weights

US/UK	*Metric*
1 oz.	30 grams (g)
2 oz.	60 g
4 oz. (1/4 lb)	125 g
5 oz. (1/3 lb)	155 g
6 oz.	185 g
7 oz.	220 g
8 oz. (1/2 lb)	250 g
10 oz.	315 g
12 oz. (3/4 lb)	375 g
14 oz.	440 g
16 oz. (1 lb)	500 g
2 lbs.	1 kg

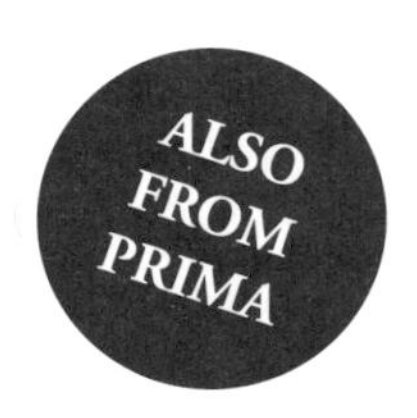

Fight Arthritis *and* Win!

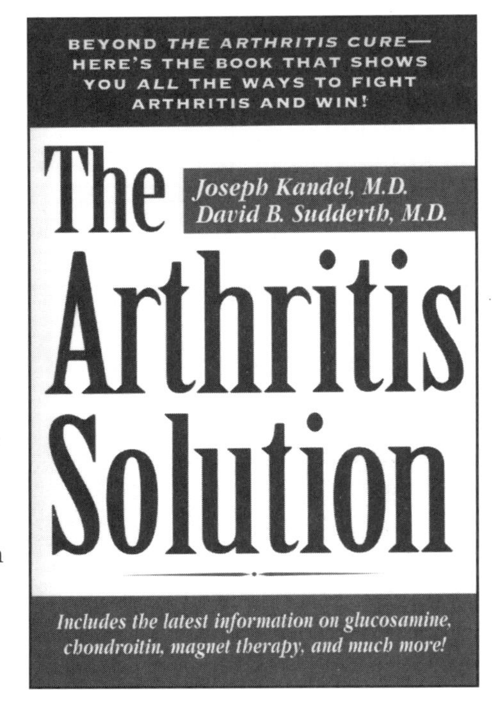

U.S. $12.00 / Can. $16.95
ISBN 0-7615-1172-5
paperback / 224 pages

Exciting new discoveries are turning osteoarthritis sufferers from helpless victims into active and victorious fighters. Now two highly respected pain specialists and neurologists show how you can relieve aching joints and possibly even reverse the impact of osteoarthritis.

The nutritional supplements glucosamine sulfate and chondroitin are the most talked-about weapons in the fight against arthritis. You'll find a full discussion of them here, along with:

- Magnet therapy
- Acupuncture
- Antioxidants
- Biofeedback
- Exercise
- Herbs and vitamins
- Ultrasound
- Physical therapy
- And much more

To order, call (800) 632-8676 or visit us online at www.primahealth.com